Keto Diet Cookbook 2020

21 Days Low Carb Ketogenic Meal Plan to Rapid Weight Loss, Have Easy Tasty Dishes, and Better Your Lifestyle (Lose Up To 21 Pounds In 3 Weeks)

Jenny C. Andy

Contents

Introduction...5

Chapter 1: Lose 1 Pound per Day with the Ketogenic Diet...7

   THE CORE ASPECTS OF BODY WEIGHT..7

   DOES A LOW-CARB KETOGENIC DIET REALLY WORK?.................................8

   BRIEF DEFINITION OF BODY NUTRIENTS...10

   A KETOGENIC DIET..10

   BENEFITS OF KETOGENIC DIET..11

   WHEN IS MY BODY IN KETOSIS?..12

   MOST IMPORTANT MISTAKES TO AVOID...12

   THE STEPS FOR SUCCESSFUL KETO WEIGHT LOSS JOURNEY....................13

Chapter 2: Mouth-watering Breakfast Recipes..14

   Protein Pancakes...14

   Almond and Coconut Mug Muffin..15

   Pineapple Smoothie..16

   Apple Muffin with Pecan Streusel..17

   Cinnamon Pie Crust With Fruit Filling..18

   Waffles...19

   Egg filled Bell Pepper Rings..20

   Baked Egg and Asparagus..21

   Breakfast Tacos..22

   Breakfast Burger...23

   Ham and Cheddar Omelet...24

   Mini Pancake Donuts..25

   Pizza Waffles..26

Chapter 3: Easy Lunch Recipes...27

   Broiled Parmesan Tilapia...27

   Blue Cheese & Bacon Stuffed Pork Chops..28

   Pan-Fried Tuna Patty...29

   Crustless Quiche Lorraine...30

   Asian Beef Salad..31

   Almond And Parmesan Crusted Tilapia...32

   Apricot Glazed Brisket..33

   Simplified Barbeque Chicken..34

   Bacon, Avocado, Chicken Sandwich...35

   Crispy Tofu And Bok Choy Salad..36

   Cheese Stuffed Bacon Wrapped Hot Dogs...37

Chicken Enchilada Soup...38

Jalapeno Popper Mug Cake...39

Thai Peanut Shrimp Curry...40

Chapter 4: Delicious Snack Recipes...41

Apricot-Apple Cloud...41

Artichoke With Three Cheeses..42

Peanut Butter Granola Bar with Strawberries And Yogurt Parfait............43

Blackberry Peach Compote..44

Baked Brie...45

Indian Chicken Curry..46

Avocado Salsa...47

Chicken Wings..48

Cauliflower Mushroom Risotto..49

Coconut Orange Creamsicle Fat Bombs...50

Corndog Muffins..51

Layered Fried Queso Blanco..52

Raspberry Lemon Popsicles...53

Neapolitan Fat Bombs...54

No Bake Chocolate Peanut Butter Balls...55

Pizza Fat Bombs...56

Sage and Cheddar Waffles...57

Chapter 5: Flavorful Dessert Recipes..58

Blueberry Mug Muffin..58

Apple Tart..59

Berries With Chocolate Ganache...60

Caramelized Pear Custard..61

Chocolate Brownie Drops...62

Baked Pear Fans...63

Chocolate Frosty..64

Ginger Flan..65

Coconut Cashew Bars..66

Choco Peanut Tart...67

Brownies..68

Mini Vanilla Cloud Cupcakes...69

Pumpkin Pecan Pie Ice Cream..70

Amaretti Cookies...71

Chocolate Dipped Macaroons...72

Chapter 6: Healthy Dinner Recipes 73

    Baked Lemon Pork Chops 73

    Cali Mac & Cheese 74

    Avocado and Cheddar Omelet 75

    Yorkshire Pudding 76

    Stuffed Red Bell Peppers 77

    Braised Leeks and Fennel 78

    Maple and Sage Pumpkin 79

    Spicy Buffalo Cauliflower 80

    Asian Short Ribs 81

    Italian Stuffed Meatballs 82

    Nacho Chicken Casserole 83

    Oven Baked Turkey Leg 84

    Slow Cooker Braised Oxtail 85

    Sushi 86

    Walnut Crusted Salmon 87

Chapter 7: Perfect Drink Recipes 88

    Blueberry Banana Smoothie 88

    Blackberry Chocolate Milkshake 89

    Cucumber Spinach Smoothie 90

    Peanut Butter Caramel Milkshake 91

    Strawberry Milkshake 92

    Tropical Smoothie 93

Chapter 8: 21-Day Keto Diet Weight Loss Meal Plan 94

    WHAT IS A MEAN PLAN? 94

    SIX BENEFITS OF HAVING A MEAL PLAN 94

    Week 1: Shopping List 94

    Week 1: Meal Plan 95

    Week 2: Shopping List 98

    Week 2: Meal Plan 99

    Week 3: Shopping List 103

    Week 3: Meal Plan 103

Conclusion 108

Congratulations and thank you for choosing this ultimate ketogenic weight loss book: "Keto Diet Cookbook 2020- 21 Days Low Carb Ketogenic Meal Plan to Rapid Weight Loss, Have Easy Tasty Dishes, and Better Your Lifestyle (Lose Up To 21 Pounds In 3 Weeks)"

Do you want to stop foods from going to fat–storing areas like your behind, belly, and thighs? Would you like to get more slender or stronger than before? **Have you considered giving up your plans of weight loss?** What if I told you that you can lose weight fast, feel better, look more beautiful or handsome, have more energy, less pain, boost your sexual prowess, keep away from disease… and most importantly, still able to eat your favorite foods and get slimmer? The Ketogenic Diet is your answer.

Learn about the core aspects of weight gain. With the ketogenic diet and you can lose one pound per day and never gain it back. Until now, most people thought it's a challenge to get rid of the fat. The methods in this book are simple, and powerful. It may sound incredible when you read it first. This Amazing Fat Destroying method will give you a total body makeover without supplements, workouts or the high price ineffective fat loss pills. It can work on anybody, no matter what weight, shape, and body type you are.

After many years of experience, everything I know was put into this book. It will slow down the aging process, and makes you look younger and more beautiful. You can benefit from it as much as I have. Prepare yourself for some astonishing results in these next few weeks.

This book was made to lead anyone from being a novice to a professional. Learn which foods to eat and which ones to avoid, help proper nourishment, and support long-lasting fat loss, anti-aging, boundless natural energy and a better mood. The book is full of powerful information that is easy to understand and designed to provide the maximum effect in minimum time.

Therefore, what are some of the benefits you get by following this program?

1. Better skin, look younger, less wrinkles and discoloration from acne

2. Rapid fat loss without exercise

3. Reduce inches from your overall body measurements

4. Sleep better and wake up easier and timely

5. Increase body energy level with no coffee or pills

6. And much more

What will you find here?

1. Essential Knowledge of Ketogenic Diet

2. The most important ketogenic diet mistakes to remember

3. Great foods that influence fat loss and your well-being

4. 80 easy and delicious recipes to keep you slimmer and healthier

5. Complete nutrition values, step-by-step procedure of each recipe

6. A 3-week rapid fat loss meal plan with healthy shopping list

Included in these 80 Ketogenic Fat Loss recipes are well-chosen and chef-proved. Each recipe has full nutrition value. It will be clearer about what your consumption of every meal to control your weight.

Welcome to the world of Ketogenic Diet for Rapid Weight Loss.

Affectionately,

Jenny C. Andy

The word Ketogenic is getting a lot of hype these days and comes to the lime light more often than before. Since the whole diet plan of our book is based on a Ketogenic lifestyle, we will dive deeper to expand your understanding of the Ketogenic Diet. However, before we touch the concept of Ketogenic Diet and how it links to weight loss, let's have a look at what our "Body Weight" is actually comprised of.

THE CORE ASPECTS OF BODY WEIGHT

These days, everybody is always talking about losing his or her weight and turning into the next hot diva or mister universe. Nevertheless, have you ever wondered what they are actually referring to? The answer is simple. By the term "Weight", they generally refer to the amount of mass on our body. That is the bulk amount coming from all the water, body fat, bones and muscle, which altogether comprises our skeletal and humanoid infrastructure.

When someone is referred to as being "Fat" or "Obese", in the simplest of terms, it is usually said they have an excess of body fat around their exterior or interior that exceeds healthy levels and is now harmful to the physical condition of a body.

More often than not, professionals such as doctors or nurses follow something called the BMI or Body Mass Index.

In the simpleton language, the BMI is a method of measure obtained by comparing the height and weight of a person to get an estimate of the person's physique. The formula below calculates the BMI of a person.

$$\text{Body Mass Index} = \frac{\text{Weight (in kg)}}{\text{Height}^2 \text{ (in m)}}$$

Once the Index is calculated, a similar chart to the one below evaluates the results.

The standards of the chart has been set by the World Health Organization who proclaim that a BMI of anywhere between 25-30 usually results in a person being overweight while 30+ would deem him/her obese.

Sadly, though, at the time of this writing, the level of people suffering from obesity and a high body fat percentage was at all-time high. In fact, in 2014 it was estimated that almost 600 million adults were suffering from obesity while 42 million of the total obese population were children under five! All thanks to the glorious fast food industry!

As a result, the next essential question in everyone's mind is "does a Ketogenic Diet or a High-Fat low Carb Diet actually help water down the level of fat? "

From the chart below, you can easily assess what category you fit under; underweight, normal, overweight or obese.

BMI CHART

12-18 Underweight   18-24 Healthy   25-29 Overweight   30-39 Obese   40-42 Extremely Obese

Weight lbs	100	105	110	115	120	125	130	135	140	145	150	155	160	165	170	175	180	185	190	195	200	205	210	215
kgs	45.5	47.7	52.3	50.0	54.5	56.8	59.1	61.4	63.6	65.9	68.2	70.5	72.7	75.0	77.3	79.5	81.8	84.1	86.4	88.6	90.9	93.2	95.5	97.7
Hight in/cm																								
5'0"-152.4	19	20	21	22	23	24	25	26	27	28	29	30	31	32	33	34	35	36	37	38	39	40	41	42
5'1"-154.9	18	19	20	21	22	23	24	25	26	27	28	29	30	31	32	33	34	35	36	36	37	38	39	40
5'2"-157.4	18	19	20	21	22	22	23	24	25	26	27	28	29	30	31	32	33	33	34	35	36	37	38	39
5'3"-160.0	17	18	19	20	21	22	23	24	24	25	26	27	28	29	30	31	32	32	33	34	35	36	37	38
5'4"-162.5	17	18	18	19	20	21	22	23	24	24	25	26	27	28	29	30	31	31	32	33	34	35	36	37
5'5"-165.1	16	17	18	19	20	20	21	22	23	24	25	25	26	27	28	29	30	30	31	32	33	34	35	35
5'6"-167.6	16	17	17	18	19	20	21	21	22	23	24	25	25	26	27	28	29	29	30	31	32	33	34	34
5'7"-170.1	15	16	17	18	18	19	20	21	22	22	23	24	25	25	26	27	28	29	29	30	31	32	32	33
5'8"-172.7	15	15	16	17	18	19	19	20	21	22	22	23	24	25	25	26	27	28	28	29	30	31	32	32
5'9"-175.2	14	15	16	17	17	18	19	20	20	21	22	22	23	24	25	25	26	27	28	28	29	30	31	31
5'10"-177.8	14	15	15	16	17	18	18	19	20	20	21	22	23	23	24	25	25	26	27	28	28	29	30	30
5'11"-180.3	14	14	15	16	16	17	18	18	19	20	21	21	22	23	23	24	25	25	26	27	28	28	29	30
5'12"-182.8	13	14	14	15	16	17	17	18	19	19	20	21	21	22	23	23	24	25	25	26	27	27	28	29
5'13"-185.4	13	13	14	15	15	16	17	17	18	19	19	20	21	21	22	23	23	24	25	25	26	27	27	28
5'14"-187.9	12	13	14	14	15	16	16	17	18	18	19	19	20	21	21	22	23	23	24	25	25	26	27	27
5'15"-190.5	12	13	13	14	15	15	15	16	17	18	18	19	20	20	21	21	22	22	23	24	25	25	26	26
5'16"-193.0	12	12	13	14	14	15	15	16	17	17	18	18	19	20	20	21	22	22	23	23	24	25	25	26

<u>DOES A LOW-CARB KETOGENIC DIET REALLY WORK?</u>

The best way to tackle this question is to elaborate the outcome of a recent test that tackled the effectiveness of various diets when it came to shedding weight.

Technically, following a proper diet does indeed prevent gaining more weight and essentially helps our body to stay healthier.

To investigate that, in recent times a team of perhaps eight research scientists had a notion to bring into contrast the effectiveness of a Ketogenic Diet with three other different forms of diet over a period of 12 months in a completely randomized control trial. The participants of this experiment included an extensive collection of 311 individuals ranging from obese people to post-menopausal women.

Group-1 comprised of 76 people instructed to consume an Ornish Diet that had just about 10% lowered down calorie in comparison to the fatty foods.

Group 2 had 79 participants who were put on a LEARN Diet which comprised of the same 10% less calories, but this time it came from the saturated fats, while 55-60% of the calorie came from the carbohydrates. The psychological and physiological activities of this group were also monitored.

Group 3 comprising of 79 people had something called the "Zone Diet" which consisted of roughly 30%, 40% and 30% distribution of calories coming from protein, carbohydrate and fats respectively.

Finally, the last group of 77 participants was treated to a low-carb "Ketogenic" diet.

For all these diets, each subject consumed only 20 grams of carbs per day for a period of 2-3 months. After which they were directed to eat 50g per day for the coming 9-10 months.

After 12 months, the result is that all diets had shown a significant amount of reduction in BMI and overall weight alongside the percentage of body fat. However, the one that showed the maximum decline was the Ketogenic diet style.

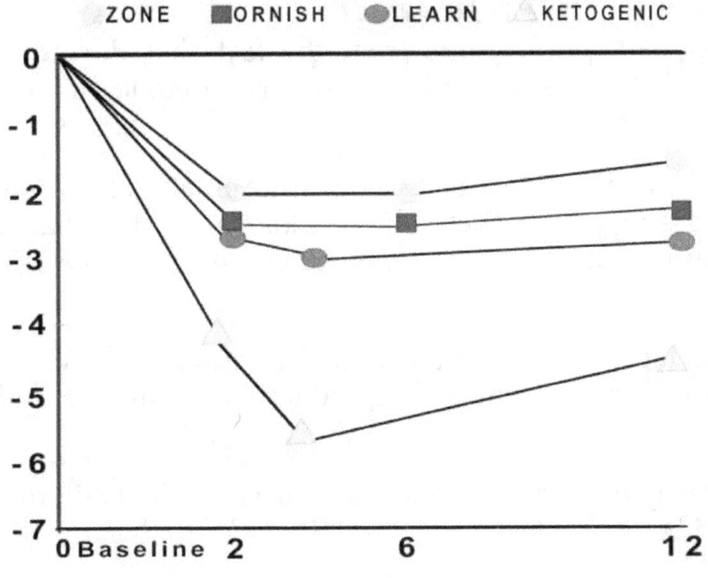

The above graph sums up the whole scenario nicely. As you can see, the decrease in BMI of the Ketogenic group is the largest. It declines a lot more than the other three diets group (LEARN group, Ornish group and Zone group).

And that's not all! Just look at the trimmed down body fat, the effects were more astonishing! The recorded decrease from the Ketogenic diet was at an astounding 7.9% while the others had a reduction of 2.5%, 2.3% and 2% in the Ornish, Zone and LEARN group respectively.

This conclusion even further supports the theory of the effectiveness of a low carb diet. In the meantime, this will help you largely to appreciate just how effective a modern Ketogenic Diet is in toning down that excess fat.

BRIEF DEFINITION OF BODY NUTRIENTS

Appreciate that our body essentially requires six nutrients and familiarize yourself with the four items below required for your Keto journey.

- **Water:** Our body is composed of almost 2/3 of water and our body needs a minimum 2 quarts of water per day to stay healthy and fit.
- **Protein:** These are the building blocks of our body. They help to generate and heal the different kind of tissues in our body. Protein promotes growth and development.
- **Fat:** Fats are often frowned upon; nevertheless, these are also essential acting as a backup reservoir of energy for the body.
- **Carbohydrates:** Carbohydrates are the primary source of energy in our body. They range from simple to complex and often converted to energy.

A KETOGENIC DIET

The primary definition of the word "Keto" results from the fact that during a specific metabolic process in our body called Ketosis, our body produces Ketones in return. The word "Keto" essentially directs toward these chemicals.

The core aim of Keto diet is to lower the levels of carbohydrate intake of the body while increasing the intake of Fat. That is why Keto Diet is largely known as High-Fat Low Carb Diet or simply Low Carb Diet. In our book, we are going to call it "Keto Diet/ Ketogenic Diet" for the sake of simplicity.

To understand how it works, the mechanism behind it shall be examined. Whenever our body is exposed to a large level of carbohydrates, the production of Glucose and Insulin tends to rise to its peak.

At this point, Glucose is a very easily convertible molecule that helps the body to normally get its energy for day-to-day activities.

Insulin acts as a companion molecule that helps to regulate the level of glucose in our blood stream. If glucose levels rise beyond normal, insulin helps to lower it. Given the fact that the body uses glucose as its core source of energy, the fat usually is not burned and stays in our bodies.

On a high carbohydrate diet, the fat levels won't come down because the body is always breaking down Carbohydrates. This is where Ketogenic Diet kicks in. By depriving your body of Carbohydrates, it automatically goes into a state known as "ketosis". Here it will release a good number of Ketones that will encourage the body to use the body fat to supply energy to the body. While in ketosis, the liver starts burning body fats as fuel. As a result, more fats are burned, more energy is produced, and you begin losing weight. It's because the fat deposits are used as a source of energy for the body.

BENEFITS OF KETOGENIC DIET

A list of Health Benefits secured from a Keto Diet will be never ending. Nevertheless, for your convenience, a few of the more important health benefits that you can gain from a Keto Diet will be explained.

- ✓ A good Ketogenic diet will help you lower the levels of bad cholesterol to prevent arterial blocks from occurring
- ✓ Energy used by burning body fat will always keep you energetic since body fat is present in abundance in our bodies
- ✓ The levels of LDL will decrease which will make the body less prone to suffer from Type-2 Diabetes
- ✓ You won't always feel hungry
- ✓ Ketosis helps improve skin conditions and prevents acne or skin inflammations from taking place.

Apart from that, you are obviously interested in knowing how a Keto Diet promotes weight loss right? Here's how:

- A Ketogenic Diet greatly increases the Protein intake which ultimately leads to weight loss promotion
- By limiting the amount of carbohydrate intake of your body, you are also restricting yourself from various foods, which will ultimately reduce the calorie intake (a key factor for weight loss) as well.
- As discussed earlier, with the process of Gluconeogenesis, the body starts to burn more fats and protein into carbs to support the body with enough energy. That itself helps to burn more calories every single day.
- The Ketogenic Diet promotes the production of appetite suppressing hormones such as Leptin and Ghrelin to reduce the feeling of hunger, allowing you to go throughout the day eating less food.
- A Ketogenic diet directly helps to increase the level of fat burnt throughout the entire day with exercise and daily activities

WHEN IS MY BODY IN KETOSIS?

Apart from being able to actually test the level of Ketones by taking samples of urine, breath or blood,certain indications will help you recognize that your body is in fact in a state of ketosis. These include:

- Your mouth will feel dry and you have an increased thirst
- The number of bathroom visits will increase as you might need to urinate more often.
- Your breath will have a slight "Fruity" smell to it.
- You will get the aforementioned sensation of low levels of hunger and increased energy.

Great, then! So, how is a person supposed to reach an optimal level of Ketosis?

It's not really as difficult as you might expect. Given that you follow a few simple rules, you will be able to thrust your body into a state of maximum Ketosis in no time!

- The first step is clearly to reduce your daily carbohydrate intake. It's better to keep it below 20 grams if possible.
- Keep the level of protein intake at moderate levels; around 70 grams if possible.
- Remember that for Ketosis to work properly, you need to maintain an ample fat intake. Make sure to eat enough fat to satisfy your body. Don't starve yourself!
- Don't have occasional snacks. Even if you are hungry; no unnecessary snacks as they might negatively affect the level of weight loss and ketosis.

MOST IMPORTANT MISTAKES TO AVOID

With everything said and done, it should be mentioned that there are some common mistakes that are made by new Keto enthusiasts.

- Since no proper definition of how much carb is actually "Low-Carb" exists, some people often tend to shoot their carb intake to a very high level while still considering that they are under "Low-Carb". The level of daily carb should be around 20-50 for optimal experience, but a maximum of 100-150g.
- It is understood that as macronutrient, protein is very important as a body building food. It improves the level of satiety and encourages fat burning. Yet, be aware of having too much protein as the excess might turn into glucose, which will once more be burned up for energy instead of fat.
- A very big mistake made by newcomers is they naturally think that lowering the level of fat alongside the carbs might increase the fat loss. That is absolutely wrong! Keep in mind that you need the fat in your body if you want to encourage the burning of fat!
- A key aspect when it comes to enhancing your ketogenic diet is to reduce the level of insulin. While on a ketogenic diet, your insulin levels will go down significantly, which helps greatly to relieve the level of bloat. Still, with that very process,

electrolytes form our body are also flushed away. Therefore, it is essential that you balance the decrease in electrolytes by having a good amount of sodium (salt) intake to make sure that your kidneys are safe and you don't have problems such as fatigue, constipation or light headache.

The only thing left now is to know what you need and going to do, to prepare yourself for the journey ahead.

<u>THE STEPS FOR SUCCESSFUL KETO WEIGHT LOSS JOURNEY</u>

- The first and foremost step is to get a carb counter guide in order to make sure that your carb intake is at desired levels.
- Open your cupboards and refrigerator and remove anything that might have a high level of carbohydrate in them, including items of whole grain.
- Restock your pantry using only low carb foods that will help you in your Keto Journey. Refer to the shopping list in the meal plan section if need be.
- Slowly and steadily give up your old habits and accept new ones that will compliment your Keto Diet
- Remember to keep plenty of drinking water nearby and always stay hydrated.
- Create and follow a strict meal plan(**Refer to Chapter 8**)

Protein Pancakes

(Prep time: 5 minutes\ Cook time: 10 minutes\ 4 servings)

Ingredients:

- 1 Tbsp vanilla whey protein
- ¼ cup almond flour
- 3 Tbsp whole grain soy flour
- 1 tsp baking powder
- 3 large sized whole eggs
- ⅓ cup cottage cheese, creamed
- Butter for Cook

Preparation:

1. In a bowl, combine almond meal, protein powder, baking powder and soy flour. Stir.
2. In a separate bowl, whisk the eggs. Add the creamed cottage cheese. Stir until combined. Add to dry ingredients. Stir until combined.
3. On a large griddle/skillet, melt butter over surface. Scoop out ¼ cup of batter. Cook 2-3 minutes per side, until golden brown.

Nutrition Values

- Calories: 191
- Fat: 9.9g
- Carbs: 4.4g
- Protein: 20g
- Dietary Fiber: 1.6g

Almond and Coconut Mug Muffin

(Prep time: 3 minutes\ Cook time: 1 minutes\ 1 serving)

Who doesn't love a filling muffin full of yummy goodness, especially if you can make it in a mug, in a minute?

Ingredients:

- 2 Tbsp almond flour
- ⅓ Tbsp Sucralose-based sweetener
- ⅓ Tbsp organic high fiber coconut flour
- ¼ tsp minced almonds
- Pinch of dried coconut
- ½ tsp Cinnamon
- ¼ tsp baking powder
- ⅛ tsp salt
- 1 large egg
- 1 tsp extra virgin olive oil

Preparation:

1. In a larger coffee mug, add the almond flour, sweetener, coconut flour, minced almond, dried coconut, cinnamon, baking powder, salt. Stir with a fork.
2. Crack in the egg. Pour in olive oil. Stir until combined.
3. Pop into the microwave. Cook for 1 minute. Cook at 15 second intervals if more time required.
4. Top with butter and more minced almond. Use a spoon to dig out the goodness.

Nutrition Values

- Calories: 207
- Fat: 16.8g
- Carbs: 3.5g
- Protein: 9.7g
- Dietary Fiber: 3g

Pineapple Smoothie

(Prep time: 5 minutes\ Cook time: 1 minutes\ 1 serving)

This pineapple smoothie will cool you down as it fills you up.

Ingredients:

- ½ cup plain yogurt
- ¼ cup fresh or frozen pineapple pieces
- 20 blanched almonds
- ½ cup almond milk

Preparation:

1. In a blender, combine yogurt, pineapple, almonds, almond milk. Blend until a smooth consistency.
2. You can add ice cubes if you want a cooler smoothie.

Nutrition Values

- Calories: 280
- Fat: 18.6g
- Carbs: 17g
- Protein: 10.8g
- Dietary Fiber: 4.2g

Apple Muffin with Pecan Streusel

(Prep time: 15 minutes\ Cook time: 25 minutes\ 8 servings)

These apple muffins are sure to be a crowd pleaser.

Ingredients:

Batter

- 1 cup almond flour
- 2 Tbsp of high fiber coconut flour, organic
- ¼ tsp salt
- 1 tsp baking powder
- 6 Tbsp granulated sugar substitute, Erythritol
- Small pinch of Stevia
- ½ tsp cinnamon
- 2 large eggs
- ¼ cup unsweetened coconut milk
- 2 tsp pure vanilla extract
- 1 apple, chopped

Streusel

- ⅔ cup almond flour
- 6 tsp cinnamon
- ⅓ tsp salt
- 2 tsp Erythritol
- ½ cup chopped pecans
- Small pinch of Stevia
- 2 Tbsp melted butter

Preparation:

Preheat oven to 350F

1. In a small bowl, combine streusel ingredients; flour, cinnamon, salt, Erythritol, stevia and pecans. Pour in the melted butter. Stir with a fork until crumble mixture forms.
2. In a large bowl, mix the almond flour, coconut flour, salt, baking powder, cinnamon, Erythritol, Stevia, and cinnamon together.
3. In a separate bowl, whisk the eggs. Add the coconut milk, and vanilla extract. Stir in the apple pieces until a batter forms.
4. Prepare a muffin tin with 8 liners.
5. Fill the muffin cups 2/3 full. Top with a tablespoon of streusel.
6. Bake 25 minutes. Stick a toothpick in muffin, if it comes out dry, muffins are ready. Cool 10 minutes in tin.

Nutrition Values

- Calories: 242
- Fat: 20.6g
- Carbs: 5.3g
- Protein: 7.5g
- Dietary Fiber: 4.2g

Cinnamon Pie Crust With Fruit Filling

(Prep time: 10 minutes\ Cook time: 30 minutes\ 4-6 servings)

This is a fantastic pie crust base to build any pie on.

Ingredients:

- ¼ tsp salt
- 1 tsp Sucralose based sweetener
- 1 tsp cinnamon
- ½ cup unsalted cold butter, cubed
- 3 servings ⅓ cup all-purpose low-carb baking mix
- 2 Tbsp tap water
- 4-6 Tbsp sugar-free fruit jam (your choice)
- 1 egg, beaten

Preparation:

1. In a food processor, combine baking mix, cinnamon, sugar substitute. Pulse 30 seconds. Add the butter. Pulse again until a coarse crumble forms.
2. Pour in water as you pulse until a dough forms. Pulse for another 30 seconds until combined.
3. Once dough is formed, transfer to plastic wrap. Wrap and form into a 3-inch disk. Chill for 30 minutes. Dust a flat surface, roll out the dough.
4. Preheat oven to 400F.
5. Cut the dough into 6-8 squares, 3 x 3, ¼ inch thick. (This is approximate based on how large you roll out the dough.) Place the dough on parchment covered cookie sheet.
6. Add 1 tablespoon of fruit jam. Dap the edges with egg wash (egg beaten in a bowl). Place a square of dough over the bottom square of dough. Press down with a fork along the edges to close. Pierce the top of dough to allow steam to escape.
7. Bake 20 minutes, until golden brown.

Nutrition Values

- Calories: 243
- Fat: 18.6g
- Carbs: 4.5g
- Protein: 18.8g
- Dietary Fiber: 2.7g

Waffles

(Prep time: 10 minutes\ Cook time: 30 minutes\ 8 servings)

A sweet treat for the morning!

Ingredients:

- 3 servings ⅓ cup all-purpose low carb baking mix
- 2 tsp baking powder
- ¼ tsp salt
- 1 packet of sucralose based sweetener
- 1 large egg
- 1 cup half and half cream
- Butter for cooking

Preparation:

1. In a large bowl, whisk the dry ingredients; baking mix, baking powder, sugar substitute, and salt together.
2. In a separate bowl, whisk the eggs and half and half together. Pour into dry ingredients. Stir until a batter forms.
3. Let the batter rest for 5 minutes to activate the baking powder.
4. Heat up your waffle maker. Brush with butter.
5. Pour ¼ to ½ cup of batter onto heated square. Close the lid. Cook approximately 10 minutes, or instructions according to your waffle iron.
6. Top with maple syrup or fruit.

Nutrition Values

- Calories: 193
- Fat: 9g
- Carbs: 5.9g
- Protein: 21.4g
- Dietary Fiber: 1.9g

Egg filled Bell Pepper Rings

(Prep time: 10 minutes\ Cook time: 5 minutes\ 1 serving)

Bell peppers are usually spicy but with the egg, it takes off the bite for a different take on breakfast.

Ingredients:

- 1 tsp extra virgin olive oil
- ½ sweet red pepper, sliced into ½ inch rings
- 2 eggs
- ¼ cup shredded mozzarella cheese, optional
- Pinch of salt and pepper
- Fruit side: ¼ a banana, ¼ a small apple, ½ a kiwi, ¼ cup raspberries

Preparation:

1. Heat the oil in a skillet. Place the red pepper rings in. Sauté one side for 2 minutes. Flip over. Crack an egg in each ring. Season with salt and pepper.
2. Add 1-2 tablespoons of water to pan. Cover with a lid. Cook for 3-5 minutes, depending on desired texture of egg.
3. Optional: top with grated cheese, cover for 1 minute to allow the cheese to melt.
4. Serve with fruit on the side.

Nutrition Values

- Calories: 361
- Fat: 20g
- Carbs: 20.1g
- Protein: 19.9g
- Dietary Fiber: 5.8g

Baked Egg and Asparagus

(Prep time: 5 minutes\ Cook time: 10 minutes\ 1 serving)

Bake an egg over a bed of asparagus; healthy fulfilling breakfast.

Ingredients:

- 4 small spears asparagus, woodsy end chopped off
- 2 eggs
- 1 Tbsp parmesan cheese
- ⅛ tsp garlic powder
- Pinch of fresh ground black pepper

Preparation:

Preheat oven to 400F
1. Grease a small oven-safe baking dish.
2. Steam the asparagus for 2 minutes.
3. Drain, rinse under cold water and pat dry.
4. Arrange the asparagus in a circle around the baking dish. Crack in 2 eggs. Season with garlic powder, pepper.
5. Bake 5 minutes. Remove from oven. Sprinkle parmesan cheese over top. Return to oven for 3 minutes.
6. Serve immediately.

Nutrition Values

- Calories: 471
- Fat: 40g
- Carbs: 5.6g
- Protein: 20.8g
- Dietary Fiber: 4g

Breakfast Tacos
(Prep time: 10 minutes\ Cook time: 15-20 minutes\ 3 servings)

Taco Tuesday for breakfast!

Ingredients:

- 1 cup shredded mozzarella cheese
- 6 eggs
- 2 Tbsp butter
- 3 strips of bacon
- ½ an avocado, thinly sliced
- ½ cup shredded cheddar cheese
- Pinch of salt and pepper

Preparation:

Preheat oven to 375F
1. Cook the bacon. Set aside.
2. You are going to make your very own cheese taco shells. Suspend a yard stick/ruler/long spoon between two items that prop it 6 inches from a counter.
3. Heat a skillet. Scoop half a cup of mozzarella cheese on the surface. Spread into a circle. Cook for 3 minutes until golden brown. Flip, cook on other side. Lift the circle of cheese off surface, drape it over yardstick/ruler. Let it cool as you cook the others and rest of ingredients.
4. In a separate bowl, whisk the eggs. Season with salt and pepper. Melt butter in a skillet. Scramble the eggs.
5. Prepare the tacos: Place a slice of bacon in cheese taco shell. Add a couple spoons of cooked egg. Top with shredded cheddar cheese and sliced avocado.

Nutrition Values

- Calories: 443
- Fat: 36.2g
- Carbs: 4.7g
- Protein: 3g
- Fiber: 1.7g
- Dietary Fiber: 25.7g

Breakfast Burger

Prep time: 5 minutes\ Cook time: 10-15 minutes\ 6 servings)

A real burger might be out of your reach but this meat packed breakfast burger won't be.

Ingredients:

- 2 cups lean ground sausage
- 1 cup shredded pepper jack cheese
- 6 slices of bacon
- 6 eggs
- 1 Tbsp of PB fit powder
- Pinch of salt and pepper

Preparation:

1. Cook the bacon, set aside.
2. In a bowl, combine the ground sausage, salt and pepper. Form palm-size patties.
3. In a separate bowl, combine PB Fit powder and 1 teaspoon of water. Stir until combined. Add a little more water for runnier consistency. Set aside.
4. Cook the sausage patties. Once cooked on both sides, cover one side with pepper jack cheese. Let it melt.
5. Cook the eggs, sunny side up or broken yolk, your preference.
6. Assemble the burgers: A sausage patty, slice of bacon, fried egg, dollop of PB fit powder. Serve immediately.

Nutrition Values:

- Calories: 655
- Fat: 56g
- Carbs: 3.5g
- Protein: 30.5g
- Fiber: 0.5g
- Net Carbs: 3g

Ham and Cheddar Omelet
(Prep time: 5 minutes\ Cook time: 20 minutes\ 5 servings)

Go for the luxury and indulge yourself with this Ham and Cheddar Chive Soufflé.

Ingredients:

- 2 ham steaks
- 1 Tbsp butter
- ½ onion, diced
- 1 garlic clove, minced
- 7 eggs
- 1 cup shredded cheddar cheese
- ½ cup heavy cream
- Pinch of salt and pepper
- 1 Tbsp freshly chives, chopped

Preparation:

Preheat oven to 400F
1. Cook the ham steak, dice into cubes.
2. In a large bowl, combine the eggs, heavy cream, salt and pepper. Whisk until combined. Add the cubed ham.
3. Using a skillet for the oven, melt the butter. Sauté onion and garlic for 2 minutes. Pour in the egg/ham mixture.
4. Bake 20 minutes, until golden brown.
5. Garnish with chopped chives.

Nutrition Values:

- Calories: 403.8
- Fats: 39.6g
- Carbs: 3.7g
- Protein: 19.6g
- Fiber: 0.2g
- Net Carbs: 3.5g

Mini Pancake Donuts

(Prep time: 5 minutes\ Cook time: 3-5 minutes \ 22 servings)

Craving a pancake and a donut? These easy to make and tasty to eat.

Ingredients:

- 6 Tbsp cream cheese
- 3 eggs
- 4 Tbsp almond flour
- 1 Tbsp coconut flour
- 1 tsp baking powder
- 1 tsp pure vanilla extract
- 4 Tbsp Erythritol
- 10 drops liquid stevia

Preparation:

1. Using a hand blender, mix the cream cheese until smooth. Add one egg at a time, Blend after each egg until fully combined.
2. In a separate bowl, combine the almond flour, coconut flour, baking powder, Erythritol. Mix well. Add the dry ingredients slowly to the cream cheese. Blend until combined. Add the vanilla, liquid stevia. Stir until a batter forms.
3. Donut maker instructions: heat canola oil. Drop in batter by tablespoon full. Cook 2 minutes, open lid, flip to other side. Cook until golden brown.
4. Donut pan instructions: grease the pan. Bake in oven at 350F for 17-20 minutes, until golden brown.
5. Cool 5 minutes.

Nutrition Values:

- Calories: 32.1
- Fat: 2.7g
- Carbs: 0.7g
- Protein: 1.4g
- Fiber: 0.3g
- Net Carbs: 0.4g

<u>**Pizza Waffles**</u>
(Prep time: 10 minutes\ Cook time: 3-5 minutes\ 2 servings)

Who doesn't love pizza! We all do. Now imagine having pizza, for breakfast.

Ingredients:

- 4 eggs
- 1 Tbsp parmesan cheese
- 3 Tbsp almond flour
- 1 Tbsp of psyllium husk powder
- 1 Tbsp bacon grease or canola oil
- 1 Tbsp baking powder
- 1 tsp italian seasoning
- 14 slices pepperoni, diced
- Pinch of salt and pepper
- ½ cup tomato sauce
- ½ cup shredded cheddar cheese

Preparation:

1. In a bowl, combine the eggs, parmesan cheese, almond flour, husk powder, bacon powder, bacon grease or oil, Italian seasoning, pepperoni, salt, and pepper. Stir until a batter forms.
2. Heat waffle maker. Lightly brush with canola oil. Pour in ¼ to ½ cup of batter. Close waffle maker. Cook 10 minutes, or until golden brown.
3. Preheat oven to broil.
4. Remove waffles. Place on baking sheet.
5. Spoon 1 tablespoon of tomato sauce over waffle. Sprinkle cheddar cheese on top.
6. Place waffles under broiler for 1-2 minutes, until cheese melts.

Nutrition Values:

- Calories: 525.5
- Fats: 41.5g
- Carbs: 10.5g
- Protein: 29g
- Fiber: 5.5g
- Net Carbs: 5.0g

Broiled Parmesan Tilapia

(Prep time: 5 minutes\ Cook time: 10 minutes\ 4-6 servings)

Fish isn't always the tastiest but adding a bit of parmesan kicks it up a notch.

Ingredients:

- 4–6 Tilapia fillets
- ½ cup finely grated parmesan cheese
- 3 Tbsp mayonnaise
- ¼ cup softened butter
- 2 Tbsp fresh lemon juice
- ¼ tsp dried basil
- ⅛ tsp onion powder
- ⅛ tsp celery salt
- ¼ tsp ground black pepper

Preparation:

Preheat oven to broil
1. Cover a baking sheet with aluminum foil.
2. In a small bowl, combine the mayonnaise, butter, lemon juice, basil, onion powder, celery salt, pepper. Stir until mixed well.
3. Place the Tilapia in a single layer on baking sheet. Cover one side of the fillets with the dressing. Place under broiler. Bake 2-4 minutes, until golden brown.
4. Pull out the pan, flip the fillets. Spread more dressing over fillets. Return to oven. Bake another 2-4 minutes, until golden.

Nutrition Values

- Calories: 224
- Fat: 12.8g
- Carbs: 0.8g
- Protein: 25.4g
- Dietary Fiber: 0.1g

Blue Cheese & Bacon Stuffed Pork Chops

(Prep time: 15 minutes\ Cook time: 20 minutes\ 2 servings)

A powerful smash flavors.

Ingredients:

- 2 butterfly pork chops (boneless)
- ¼ cup crumbled blue cheese
- 2 slices of bacon, cooked, crumbled
- 2 Tbsp fresh chives, chopped
- Pinch of garlic powder
- Pinch of fresh ground black pepper
- Fresh parsley, garnish

Preparation:

Preheat oven to 325F
1. Slice pork chops length-wise to create a pocket.
2. Grease a shallow baking dish with butter.
3. In a small bowl, combine the blue cheese, chives, and bacon. Mix well.
4. Divide mixture in half, roll loosely into balls.
5. Place a ball in the pocket of each butterflied pork chop. Close with a toothpick.
6. Season both sides of pork chops with garlic salt, and pepper.
7. Bake 20 minutes, until pork chops are cooked through. Flip pork chops halfway through cooking. (Pork internal temperature: 165F)
8. Remove from oven. Cover with foil and rest for 5 minutes (will allow the dressing inside to settle.) Garnish with fresh parsley.

Nutrition Values

- Calories: 394
- Fat: 26.3g
- Carbs: 2g
- Protein: 36g
- Dietary Fiber: 0.3g

Pan-Fried Tuna Patty

(Prep time: 15 minutes\ Cook time: 5 minutes\ 2 servings)

Everybody loves Tuna! Now you can enjoy it as a burger.

Ingredients:

- 1 can of tuna packed in water
- 1 egg
- ½ stalk of celery, chopped
- 2 Tbsp chopped walnuts
- 2 Tbsp fresh parsley, chopped
- 1 tsp fresh dill, chopped
- Pinch of salt and pepper
- 2 Tbsp mayonnaise
- 1 Tbsp butter
- ¼ cup shredded cheddar cheese

Preparation:

1. Drain the water from can of tuna.
2. In a bowl, combine tuna, egg, celery, chopped walnut, parsley, dill, salt, and pepper. Stir until fully combined. Add the mayonnaise. Stir again to mix.
3. Divide mixture in half. Form two round patties.
4. In a skillet, melt the butter. Cook the patties 2 minutes, flip to other side.
5. Sprinkle shredded cheese on cooked side. Cook patty another 2 minutes.
6. Serve immediately.

Nutrition Values

- Calories: 367
- Fat: 29.3g
- Carbs: 2.4g
- Protein: 24.2g
- Dietary Fiber: 0.8g

<u>**Crustless Quiche Lorraine**</u>
(Prep time: 10 minutes\ Cook time: 210 minutes\ 8 servings)

It might sound weird but give it a chance. This quiche may just surprise you.

Ingredients:

- 4 eggs
- 1 x 8 oz container sour cream
- 1 package frozen spinach, defrosted, drained, chopped
- 1 cup shredded cheese (mild, or sharp)
- ½ cup crumbled feta cheese
- ½ cup shredded parmesan cheese
- 1 onion, diced
- 1 tomato, diced
- ½ cup green chilies, drained, chopped
- 1 garlic clove, minced up tsp of garlic
- 1 tsp ground cumin
- 1 Tbsp paprika
- ¼ tsp cayenne pepper

Preparation:

Preheat oven to 325Fahrenheit
1. In a medium bowl, add the eggs. Beat them. Whisk in the sour cream until a smooth consistency.
2. Add the cheddar cheese, parmesan cheese, feta cheese, tomato, spinach, onion, green chilies, cumin, garlic, cayenne pepper, and paprika. Stir well.
3. Grease a pie plate. Pour in the batter. Place the pie plate on a baking sheet.
4. Bake 1 hour. Allow to set 5 minutes before slicing.

Nutrition Values

- Calories: 401
- Fat: 32.4g
- Carbs: 10.6g
- Protein: 19.3g
- Dietary Fiber: 2.5g

Asian Beef Salad

(Prep time: 6-10 hours, 20 minutes\ Cook time: 5 minutes\ 1 serving)

The Asian beef salad is perfect for Ketogenic diet.

Ingredients:

- 1 small garlic clove, minced
- ½ Tbsp tamari soy sauce
- ¼ Tbsp sodium/sugar-free rice wine vinegar
- ¼ tsp sesame oil
- ⅛ tsp based sweetener
- ⅛ tsp curry powder
- Pinch of ground ginger
- 4 pieces ¼ ounce beef top sirloin
- ½ Tbsp canola oil
- ¾ cup spring mixed salad greens
- 1 small red bell pepper
- ¼ cup water chestnuts, sliced
- 1 scallion, diced
- Asian dressing

Preparation:

1. In a Ziploc bag, combine minced garlic, soy sauce, rice wine vinegar, sesame oil, sugar, curry powder, ginger. Add steak to bag. Massage steak through bag to coat.
2. Place in the fridge to marinate over night.
3. The next day, remove the steak from the bag. (Discard the marinade.) Set on a plate to bring to room temperature before cooking, approximately 30 minutes.
4. Heat the oil in a skillet. Place the steak in the skillet. Cook 5-6 minutes per side.
5. Remove from pan. Let the steak rest 10 minutes before slicing.
6. In a large bowl, add the mixed salad greens, red bell pepper, water chest nuts, and scallion.
7. Slice the steak. Add to bowl. Drizzle in Asian dressing. Toss lightly. Serve.

Nutrition Values

- Calories: 295
- Fat: 13.3g
- Carbs: 10.4g
- Protein: 29.5g
- Dietary Fiber: 4.1g

Almond And Parmesan Crusted Tilapia

(Prep time: 10 minutes\ Cook time: 10 minutes\ 4 servings)

A crunchy fish sure to tempt any pallet.

Ingredients:

- 1 tsp olive oil
- 3 garlic cloves, minced
- ½ cup grated parmesan
- ¼ cup crushed almonds
- 2 Tbsp bread crumbs
- 1 tsp seafood seasoning
- ¼ tsp dried basil
- ¼ tsp ground black pepper
- ⅛ tsp celery salt
- ¼ cup buttery spread, softened
- 3 Tbsp reduced fat olive oil mayonnaise
- 2 Tbsp fresh lemon juice
- 4 tilapia fillets

Preparation:

Adjust oven rack to 6 inches from broiler. Preheat broiler
1. Line a baking dish with aluminum foil. Lightly grease the foil.
2. In a small skillet, heat olive oil. Sauté garlic for 3 minutes. Transfer to a bowl.
3. In the bowl, also add parmesan cheese, crushed almonds, bread crumbs, seafood seasoning, basil, pepper, celery salt. Whisk to combine. Stir in buttery spread and mayonnaise until combined. Add lemon juice. Stir until mixed in well.
4. Place tilapia fillets on aluminum foil covered baking dish.
5. Place under broiler. Cook 3 minutes. Flip to other side, cook another 3 minutes.
6. Remove from oven. Spread coating on 1 side. Return to broiler. Cook 3 minutes.
7. Remove from oven. Spread coating to other side. Return to broiler. Cook 3 minutes. Fish should be flaky, and coating golden brown. Serve hot

Nutrition Values

- Calories: 344
- Fat: 21.9g
- Carbs: 6.6g
- Protein: 29.3g
- Dietary Fiber: 0.9g

Apricot Glazed Brisket

(Prep time: 15 minutes\ Cook time: 5 minutes\ 4 servings)

With this glazed Apricot Brisket, you will have no trouble winning the heart of everyone.

Ingredients:

- 2 Tbsp canola oil
- 4 pounds beef brisket
- 2 tsp salt
- 2 tsp paprika
- 1 tsp black pepper
- 2 large carrots, diced in chunks
- 1 large onion, diced in chunks
- 3 Tbsp sugar-free apricot

Preparation:

Preheat oven to 375F
1. Combine salt, pepper, paprika in a bowl. Stir until combined.
2. Spread over surface of brisket.
3. Drizzle oil over bottom of Dutch oven or pot for oven. Sear on all sides.
4. Once done, turn over brisket with fat side up. Add ½ a cup of water to pan.
5. Add carrots and onion to pan. Cook for 3-4 hours until the brisket is tender.
6. Remove brisket from oven. Spread apricot jelly over brisket. Return to oven.
7. Broil 6 inches from heat for 5 minutes until the apricot jam creates a crust.
8. Remove from oven. Cover in aluminum foil. Let it rest 15 minutes before slicing.
9. Transfer to platter. Place carrots and onions on platter or discard.

Nutrition Values

- Calories: 358
- Fat: 16g
- Carbs: 1.3g
- Protein: 47g
- Dietary Fiber: 0.3g

Simplified Barbeque Chicken
(Prep time: 10 minutes\ Cook time: 90 minutes\ 6 servings)

This recipe is designed to make the process of BBQ-ing your chicken as easy as possible.

Ingredients:

- 6 bone-in chicken breast halves, skin on
- 1 Tbsp Worcestershire sauce
- 1 Tbsp hickory flavored liquid smoke
- 2 tsp chili powder
- 2 tsp ground cumin
- 2 tsp garlic powder
- 2 tsp dried thyme
- 2 tsp dried oregano
- Pinch of salt and pepper

Preparation:

Preheat oven to 375F
1. Lightly grease 9 x 13 baking dish. Place chicken in single layer.
2. In a bowl, combine the Worcestershire sauce, liquid smoke, chili powder, cumin, garlic powder, thyme, oregano, salt, and pepper.
3. Spread coating over pieces of chicken.
4. Cover with aluminum foil. Bake for 90 minutes.
5. Serve immediately.

Nutrition Values

- Calories: 330
- Fat: 14g
- Carbs: 2.6g
- Protein: 45.4g
- Dietary Fiber: 0.9g

Bacon, Avocado, Chicken Sandwich

(Prep time: 10 minutes\ Cook time: 25 minutes\ 2 servings)

Boot up your system after a long day with this hearty chicken, bacon, avocado on cloud bread sandwich.

Ingredients:

Cloud Bread

- 3 eggs
- ¼ cup cream of tartar
- ¼ cup cream cheese
- ¼ tsp salt
- ½ tsp garlic powder

Filling

- 1 Tbsp mayonnaise
- 1 tsp siracha
- 2 slices of bacon
- 1 chicken breast fillet
- 2 slices pepper jack cheese
- ¼ avocado, sliced

Preparation:

Preheat oven to 300F
1. Separate the eggs in to 2 different bowls.
2. Bowl with egg whites, add cream of tartar. Blend with electric mixer until fluffy.
3. Bowl with egg yolks, add cream cheese. Blend with electric mixer until smooth.
4. Slowly fold the fluffy egg whites in to egg yolk mixture.
5. Line a baking sheet with parchment paper.
6. Scoop ¼ cups of batter on baking sheet.
7. Smooth batter in to a circle. Sprinkle salt and garlic powder over clouds.
8. Bake 25 minutes.
9. While cloud bread is baking, in a skillet, cook the bacon, then the chicken. Season chicken breast with salt and pepper. Slice chicken breast after cooked.
10. Remove clouds from oven. Remove with a flipper to a flat surface.
11. Slice the avocado.
12. Combine mayonnaise and siracha sauce in a bowl. Stir until combined.
13. Spread a layer of spicy mayo on one cloud bread.
14. Place a slice of pepper jack cheese, then chicken, slice of bacon. Top with another cloud bread.

Nutrition Values:

- Calories: 361
- Fat: 28.25g
- Carbs: 4g
- Protein: 2g
- Fiber: 2g
- Net Carbs: 22g

Crispy Tofu And Bok Choy Salad

(Prep time: 6-7 hours, 20 minutes \ Cook time: 30-35 minutes\ 3 servings)

Tofu and Bok Choy to give you a hearty new take on tofu. Don't knock it 'til you try it.

Ingredients:

Oven baked tofu

- 1 cup extra firm tofu
- 1 Tbsp soy sauce
- 1 Tbsp sesame oil
- 1 Tbsp of water
- 2 garlic cloves, minced
- 1 Tbsp rice wine vinegar
- Juice from ½ a lemon

Bok Choy Salad

- 6 heads baby Bok Choy
- 1 green onion, diced
- 2 Tbsp cilantro, chopped
- 3 Tbsp coconut oil, heated in microwave and cooled
- 2 Tbsp soy sauce
- 1 Tbsp sambal olek
- 1 Tbsp natural peanut butter
- Juice from ½ a lime
- 2 drops liquid stevia

Preparation:

1. Wrap the tofu in a clean tea towel. Place a heavy pot/cast iron skillet on top. Press out moisture for 6 hours. Swap out tea towel for dry one at halfway point.
2. Once dried out, slice into cubes.
3. In a bowl, combine soy sauce, sesame oil, water, minced garlic, rice wine vinegar, lemon juice. Stir well. Pour marinade in large Ziploc bag. Add tofu cubes. Massage tofu through bag to coat. Marinate in fridge 30 minutes to 8 hours.
4. When ready to cook. Preheat oven to 350F. Place tofu on parchment covered baking sheet in a single layer. Bake 35 minutes.
5. As it bakes, in a bowl, combine the coconut oil, soy sauce, sambal olek, peanut butter, lime juice, stevia. Stir until combined.
6. Chop up the Bok Choy. Add the diced green onion, and cilantro.
7. Remove tofu from oven.
8. Add to bowl with Bok Choy salad. Drizzle dressing over ingredients. Serve.

Nutrition Values:

- Calories: 442.3
- Fat: 35.0g
- Carbs: 7.3g
- Protein: 25.0g
- Fiber: 1.7g
- Net Carbs: 5.7g

Cheese Stuffed Bacon Wrapped Hot Dogs

(Prep time: 5-10 minutes\ Cook time: 35-40 minutes\ 6 servings)

Sometimes you just really need a guilty pleasure.

Ingredients:

- 6 all beef hot dogs
- 12 slices of bacon
- 3 slices cheddar cheese, cut in half
- ½ tsp garlic powder
- ½ tsp onion powder
- Pinch of salt and pepper

Preparation:

Preheat oven to 300F
1. Slice the hot dogs down the middle. Place sliced cheese in middle.
2. Wrap bacon around the hot dog; might take 2 slices.
3. Secure with toothpick on each end.
4. Place on baking sheet lined with parchment paper.
5. Bake 35-40 minutes, until bacon crispy.

Nutrition Values:

- Calories: 379.7
- Fat: 34.5g
- Carbs: 0.3g
- Protein: 16.8g
- Fiber: 0g
- Net Carbs: 0.3g

Chicken Enchilada Soup

(Prep time: 10 minutes\ Cook time: 30-35 minutes\ 4 servings)

An enchilada in a soup. It is good. Trust me.

Ingredients:

- 3 Tbsp olive oil
- 1 onion, diced
- 2 garlic cloves, minced
- 3 stalks of celery, sliced
- 1 red bell pepper, diced
- 1 cup diced tomatoes
- 4 cups of chicken broth
- 1 package 8-ounce cream cheese
- ½ cup cooked chicken breast or thigh, shredded
- 2 tsp cumin
- 1 tsp oregano
- 1 tsp chili powder
- ½ tsp cayenne pepper
- Juice from ½ a lime
- Cilantro for garnish
- Shredded cheddar cheese, garnish

Preparation:

1. In a large skillet, heat the olive oil. Sauté the onion, garlic, red pepper, and celery for 5 minutes.
2. Add the tomatoes. Stir and cook for 3 minutes. Add the cumin, oregano, chili powder, cayenne pepper. Stir again.
3. Pour in the chicken broth and stir. Simmer for 10 minutes.
4. After 10 minutes, stir in the cream cheese. Simmer on low heat 5 minutes.
5. Add shredded cooked chicken. Stir. Simmer 5 minutes. Squeeze in the lime juice.
6. Serve in bowls. Garnish with cilantro and shredded cheese.

Nutrition Values:

- Calories: 344.8
- Fat: 31.3g
- Carbs: 7.8g
- Protein: 13.3g
- Fiber: 1.8g
- Net Carbs: 6.0g

Jalapeno Popper Mug Cake

(Prep time: 5 minutes\ Cook time: 10-15 minutes\ 1 serving)

If you have what it takes to survive the spiciness of jalapeno!

Ingredients:

- 2 Tbsp almond flour
- 1 Tbsp golden flaxseed
- ½ tsp baking powder
- Pinch of salt and pepper
- 1 slice of bacon
- ½ a jalapeno pepper
- 1 egg
- 1 Tbsp butter
- 1 Tbsp cream cheese

Preparation:

1. Cook the bacon.
2. In a mug, combine the almond flour, flaxseed, baking powder, salt, pepper, bacon, jalapeno pepper. Stir everything.
3. Beat the egg slightly. Pour into mug. Stir it in.
4. Add the butter, cream cheese. Stir.
5. Microwave for 75 seconds, on power 10.
6. Fork or spoon, eat it right out of the mug.

Nutrition Values:

- Calories: 429
- Fat: 38g
- Carbs: 8.4g
- Protein: 16.5g
- Fiber: 4.2g
- Net Carbs: 4.2g

Thai Peanut Shrimp Curry

(Prep time: 10 minutes\ Cook time: 10-20 minutes\ 2 servings)

Have a bowl of rice but nothing to go with? Cook up a batch of Thai Shrimp.

Ingredients:

- 2 Tbsp coconut oil
- 1 spring onion, diced
- 1 garlic clove, crushed
- ½ tsp turmeric
- ¼ cup broccoli florets
- 2 Tbsp green curry paste
- 1 Tbsp soy sauce
- 1 Tbsp peanut butter
- 1 tsp fish sauce
- 1 cup vegetable broth
- 1 cup coconut milk
- 3 Tbsp chopped cilantro
- ¼ tsp xanthan gum
- ½ cup cream
- 1 cup pre-cooked shrimp
- Juice from ½ a lime

Preparation:

1. In a large skillet, heat the coconut oil. Sauté the minced ginger and spring onion for 1 minute. Add the turmeric and curry paste.
2. Stir in the soy sauce, peanut butter, and fish sauce. Mix them well.
3. Pour in vegetable broth and coconut milk. Add the broccoli. Simmer 5 minutes.
4. Stir in xanthan gum and cream. Add the shrimp. Simmer 10 minutes.
5. Serve over rice. Squirt lime juice over the curry.

Nutrition Values:

- Calories: 454.5g
- Fat: 31.5g
- Carbs: 13.7g
- Protein: 27g
- Fiber: 4.8g
- Net Carbs: 8.9g

Apricot-Apple Cloud

(Prep time: 65 minutes\ Cook time: 10 minutes\ 6 servings)

Even though the apricot apple cloud seems geared towards children, don't let it fool you. It is a snack worthy of any Ketogenic Diet follower.

Ingredients:

- 1½ cups heavy cream
- 2 cups unsweetened applesauce baby food
- 2 Tbsp sucralose based sweetener

Preparation:

1. In a large bowl, using an electric mixer, whip the heavy cream. Add the sugar substitute. Beat until firm peaks form.
2. Gently fold in applesauce. Stir until combined.
3. Pour into 6 individual serving bowls.
4. Chill for 1 hour. Serve.

Nutrition Values

- Calories: 9.9
- Fat: 22.4
- Carbs: 25g
- Protein: 1.5g
- Dietary Fiber: 1.1g

Artichoke With Three Cheeses

(Prep time: 20 minutes\ Cook time: 40 minutes\ 4 servings)

Yet another intelligent way to get you to eat your green vegetable. Try not to gobble it.

Ingredients:

- 2 cups artichoke hearts
- ½ cup vegetable broth
- 3 Tbsp extra virgin olive oil
- 1 tsp lemon juice
- 2 garlic cloves, minced
- Fresh parsley, chopped
- Fresh basil, chopped
- ½ cup shredded Fontina cheese
- ½ cup of shredded Swiss cheese
- ½ cup shredded Parmesan cheese

Preparation:

Preheat oven to 400F
1. Arrange artichokes in single layer of a deep baking dish.
2. Drizzle oil, lemon juice, garlic, vegetable broth over the artichokes.
3. Start with fontina cheese, then Swiss cheese, parmesan cheese last.
4. Cover baking dish with aluminum foil. Bake 15 minutes.
5. Remove foil. Bake an additional 15 minutes, until cheese is golden and bubbly.
6. Remove from oven. Let it cool to room temperature. Serve.

Nutrition Values

- Calories: 57
- Fat: 14g
- Carbs: 3g
- Protein: 4g
- Dietary Fiber: 2.6g

Peanut Butter Granola Bar with Strawberries And Yogurt Parfait

(Prep time: 5 minutes\ Cook time: 0 minutes\ 1 serving)

Granola bars are an excellent source of energy and combined with yogurt and strawberries, they can turn into a great ketogenic suitable snack.

Ingredients:

- 1 cup plain Greek yogurt
- 1 Ketogenic Peanut Butter Granola Bar
- 5 strawberries, sliced

Preparation:

1. Place the granola bar in a baggie. Break up into small pieces.
2. Spoon a layer of yogurt in bottom of a dish.
3. Add a layer of smashed granola bar.
4. Spoon in a layer of yogurt.
5. Top with strawberries.
6. Serve immediately or chill in refrigerator.

Nutrition Values

- Calories: 314
- Fat: 9.5g
- Carbs: 12.6g
- Protein: 24.1g
- Dietary Fiber: 6.8g

Blackberry Peach Compote

(Prep time: 10 minutes\ Cook time: 20 minutes\ 12 servings)

This can be considered as both a snack and a desert.

Ingredients:

- ¼ cup Sauvignon Blanc wine
- 2 Tbsp Xylitol
- 1 tsp ground ginger
- 1 tsp Cinnamon
- 3 medium peaches
- ¼ cup blackberries
- ½ tsp thick it up

Preparation:

1. In a large saucepan, combine the wine, Xylitol, ginger, peaches, and cinnamon.
2. Simmer for 15 minutes.
3. Add the blackberries. Simmer another 5 minutes, until berries are tender.
4. Stir in the thick it up. Simmer approximately 5 minutes.
5. Remove from heat. Cool to room temperature. Serve.

Nutrition Values

- Calories: 35
- Fat: 0.2g
- Carbs: 4.2g
- Protein: 0.5g
- Dietary Fiber: 3.4g

Baked Brie
(Prep time: 5 minutes\ Cook time: 10 minutes\ 6 servings)

Melted cheese. Who could resist?

Ingredients:

- 8 oz Brie wheel cheese
- ¼ cup pine nuts

Preparation:

Heat oven to 450F
1. Trip top of white rind off cheese.
2. Cover top with pine nuts.
3. Place cheese on aluminum foil pan or pie dish.
4. Bake 10 minutes. Serve.

Nutrition Values

- Calories: 144
- Fat: 12.1g
- Carbs: 2.g
- Protein: 8.2g
- Dietary Fiber: 0.1g

Indian Chicken Curry

(Prep time: 8 minutes\ Cook time: 20 minutes\ 6 servings)

This curry is designed to give you the flavor of core Indian curries.

Ingredients:

- 3 Tbsp unsalted butter
- 2 garlic cloves, minced
- 4 chicken breasts, boneless, skinless
- 1 tsp cumin
- ½ tsp coriander
- ½ tsp ground ginger
- ¼ tsp crushed red pepper flakes
- ½ cup chicken broth
- ⅓ cup heavy cream
- Fresh cilantro

Preparation:

1. In a large skillet, melt the butter. Sauté the garlic for 2 minutes.
2. Add the chicken breasts. Cook thoroughly.
3. Once cooked, remove the chicken and cut into chunks. Return to the pan.
4. Pour in the chicken broth, cumin, coriander, ginger, red pepper flakes.
5. Turn down the heat to medium-low. Simmer 5 minutes.
6. Stir in the cream. Simmer another 3 minutes.
7. Serve in bowls over rice. Garnish with fresh cilantro.

Nutrition Values

- Calories: 413
- Fat: 22.1g
- Carbs: 1g
- Protein: 49.1g
- Dietary Fiber: 0.3g

Avocado Salsa

(Prep time: 10 minutes\ Cook time: 0 minutes\ 4 servings)

Avocados are really great, turning it into a salsa, even greater.

Ingredients:

- 1 red tomato
- ⅛ cup fresh cilantro, rough chopped
- 1 red onion, diced
- ½ jalapeno pepper, diced
- 2 avocadoes, diced
- 2-3 Tbsp fresh lime juice
- Pinch of salt and fresh ground black pepper

Preparation:

1. Chop all the vegetables.
2. Add them to a bowl.
3. Squeeze in the lime juice. Season with salt and pepper. Stir.
4. Refrigerate for 30 minutes. Serve.

Nutrition Values

- Calories: 71
- Fat: 5.3g
- Carbs: 3.3g
- Protein: 1.1g
- Dietary Fiber: 3g

Chicken Wings

(Prep time: 10 minutes\ Cook time: 35 minutes\ 8 servings)

A delicious treat.

Ingredients:

- ½ serving all purpose low carb baking mix
- 2 Tbsp chili powder
- 1 tsp cayenne pepper
- 2 tsp yellow mustard seed
- 2 tsp salt
- 12-16 chicken wings

Preparation:

Preheat oven to 450F
1. Rinse the chicken wings.
2. Line a baking sheet with aluminum foil. Spray with non-stick cooking spray.
3. Take a Ziploc bag, add the baking mix, chili powder, cayenne pepper, mustard seed, salt. Place the wings in the bag. Massage the chicken wings through the bag to coat them with seasoning.
4. Transfer to baking sheet. Cook 30-35 minutes, until golden brown.
5. Serve immediately.

Nutrition Values

- Calories: 276
- Fat: 18.5g
- Carbs: 3.4g
- Protein: 22.4g
- Dietary Fiber: 0.3g

Cauliflower Mushroom Risotto

(Prep time: 10 minutes\ Cook time: 10 minutes\ 2 servings)

A unique Italian dish with the warm flavors of mushroom and cauliflower, and healthy.

Ingredients:

- 1 Tbsp olive oil
- 2 garlic cloves, minced
- 4 baby bella mushrooms, diced
- 1 cup chicken broth
- 2 cups riced cauliflower
- ¼ cup parmesan cheese
- ¼ cup heavy cream
- 1 tsp tarragon
- Pinch of salt and pepper

Preparation:

1. In a blender, process the cauliflower until rice-like consistency.
2. In a skillet, heat the olive oil. Sauté the garlic, mushrooms for 3 minutes.
3. Pour in the chicken broth and cauliflower. Stir well. Simmer 5 minutes.
4. Once the liquid has cooked away, add the parmesan cheese and tarragon, salt, and pepper. Stir well. Stir in the cream. Keep stirring until the cheese has melted.
5. Serve hot.

Nutrition Values:

- Calories: 245.5
- Fat: 20g
- Carbs: 8.5g
- Protein: 7g
- Fiber: 2.5g
- Net Carbs: 6g

Coconut Orange Creamsicle Fat Bombs

(Prep time: 2-3 hours\ Cook time: nil\ 10 Fat bombs)

Enjoy a savory combination of coconut and orange in this fat bomb recipe.

Ingredients:

- ½ cup coconut oil
- ½ cup heavy whipping cream
- ¼ cup cream cheese
- 1 tsp orange vanilla Mio
- 10 drops liquid Stevia

Preparation:

1. Add the coconut oil to a blender. Pulse until smooth.
2. Add the whip cream. Pulse until combined.
3. Add the cream cheese. Pulse until smooth.
4. Add the orange Milo and Stevia. Pulse until smooth.
5. Spoon the mixture into silicon tray mold or ice cube tray. Freeze 3 hours.
6. Pop out to eat. Store uneaten bombs in a bag in the freezer.

Nutrition Values:

- Calories: 176
- Fat: 20g
- Carbs: 0.7g
- Protein: 0.8g
- Fiber: 0g
- Net Carbs: 0.7g

Corndog Muffins

(Prep time: 10 minutes \ Cook time: 15 minutes\ 20 Muffins)

Turn your ordinary muffin into a delightful meaty combination with these cute muffins.

Ingredients:

- ½ cup blanched almond flour
- ½ cup flaxseed meal
- 1 Tbsp psyllium husk powder
- 3 Tbsp swerve sweetener
- ¼ tsp salt
- ¼ tsp baking powder
- ¼ cup melted butter
- 1 egg
- ¼ cup coconut milk
- ⅓ cup sour cream
- 3 all beef hot dogs

Preparation:

Preheat oven to 375F

1. In a bowl, add the almond flour, flaxseed, husk powder, granulated sweetener, salt, and baking powder. Whisk together.
2. In a separate bowl, combine the egg, coconut milk. Whisk together. Add the butter. Stir until combined. Add the sour cream. Stir until combined.
3. Add the dry ingredients to the wet ingredients. Stir until a smooth batter forms.
4. Grease a 12 mini muffin tin.
5. Slice the hot dogs into 4 sections.
6. Fill the muffin cup half way. Add the sliced hot dog to the batter.
7. Bake 12 minutes.
8. Then broil 1-2 minutes, until golden brown. Serve.

Nutrition Values:

- Calories: 78.5
- Fat: 6.8g
- Carbs: 2.1g
- Protein: 2.4g
- Fiber: 1.5g
- Net Carbs: 0.7g

Layered Fried Queso Blanco

(Prep time: 10 minutes \ Cook time: 10 minutes\ multiple Servings)

Think frying up your cheese might be a bad idea? Think again.

Ingredients:

- ½ cup Queso Blanco
- 1½ Tbsp olive oil
- Pinch red pepper flakes or salt and pepper

Preparation:

1. Cut the cheese into cubes. Chill in the freezer as you heat the oil.
2. In a skillet, heat the olive oil. Once the pan is hot, add the cubes of cheese.
3. As it cooks it will melt. Once it is golden brown on one side, flip it over. Press down against the cheese to flatten it slightly and push out the oil. Once it is golden brown on both sides, tilt the edges against the pan and cook those until golden brown. It will seal the cheese into a square.
4. Remove from pan. Place on paper towel. Pat lightly. Slice into cubes again.
5. Sprinkle red pepper flakes or salt and pepper over the cubes. Serve immediately.

Nutrition Values:

- Calories: 525
- Fat: 43g
- Carbs: 4g
- Protein: 30g
- Fiber: 2g
- Net Carbs: 2g

Raspberry Lemon Popsicles

(Prep time: 10-15 minutes\ Cook time: 2 hours\ 6 servings)

How about a refreshing ice cream now?

Ingredients:

- 1 cup of raspberries
- Juice from ½ a lemon
- ¼ cup coconut oil
- 1 cup coconut milk
- ¼ cup sour cream
- ¼ cup heavy cream
- ½ tsp Guar Gum
- 20 drops liquid Stevia

Preparation:

1. Combine all the ingredients in a blender. Pulse until smooth. Strain the liquid.
2. Pour mixture into popsicle molds. Freeze 2 hours.
3. If stuck, run the mold under hot water briefly.

Nutrition Values:

- Calories: 150.5
- Fat: 16.0g
- Carbs: 3.3g
- Protein: 0.5
- Fiber: 1.3g
- Net Carbs: 2.0g

Neapolitan Fat Bombs

(Prep time: 15-30 minutes\ Cook time: 1 hour\ 24 servings)

Try out this recipe to satisfy a sweet craving.

Ingredients:

- ½ cup butter
- ½ cup coconut oil
- ½ cup sour cream
- ½ cup cream cheese
- 2 Tbsp liquid stevia
- 2 Tbsp cocoa powder
- 1 tsp pure vanilla extract
- 2 strawberries

Preparation:

1. In a blender, add the butter, coconut oil, sour cream, cream cheese. Pulse until smooth.
2. Set out 3 bowls. Add cocoa powder to a bowl. Add vanilla extract to another bowl. Add strawberries to a bowl. Mash them.
3. Pour the mixture evenly between the 3 bowls. Stir each mixture until smooth.
4. Pour vanilla mixture into bottom of silicon mold or ice cube tray. Freeze for 30 minutes. Place other bowls in the fridge. Pour the chocolate layer in the silicon mold or ice cube tray. Freeze 30 minutes. Pour the strawberry layer into the silicon mold or ice cube tray. Freeze 2 hours. Ready to serve.

Nutrition Values:

- Calories: 102.2
- Fat: 10.9g
- Carbs: 0.6g
- Protein: 0.6g
- Fiber: 0.2g
- Net Carbs: 0.4g

No Bake Chocolate Peanut Butter Balls

(Prep time: 20 minutes \ Cook time: nil\ 8 Fat bombs)

Don't even try to resist this treat.

Ingredients:

- ¼ cup cocoa powder
- 4 Tbsp Peanut Butter Fit Powder
- 5 Tbsp shelled hemp seeds
- 2 Tbsp heavy cream
- ½ cup coconut oil
- 1 tsp pure vanilla extract
- 28 drops liquid stevia
- ¼ cup unsweetened shredded coconut

Preparation:

1. In a bowl, crush the hemp seeds. Add the cocoa powder, fit powder. Stir. Add the coconut oil. Stir together until a paste forms.
2. Stir in the heavy cream, liquid stevia, and vanilla. Keep mixing until it forms a dough consistency.
3. Pinch off dough to make 1 inch round balls. Roll in unsweetened shredded coconut. Chill 30 minutes. Serve.

Nutrition Values:

- Calories: 208.3
- Fat: 20.0g
- Carbs: 3.1g
- Protein: 4.4g
- Fiber: 2.4g
- Net Carbs: 0.8g

Pizza Fat Bombs

(Prep time: 10 minutes\ Cook time: nil\ 6 Fat Bombs)

Why not fulfill your macronutrient needs by savoring pizza flavored fat bombs.

Ingredients:

- ¼ cup cream cheese
- 12 slices of pepperoni
- 6 pitted black olives
- 2 Tbsp sun dried tomato pesto
- 2 Tbsp fresh basil, chopped
- Pinch of salt and pepper

Preparation:

1. Dice up the pepperoni. Dice the black olives.
2. In a bowl, combine the cream cheese and tomato pesto. Stir in the pepperoni, black olives, and basil. Mash it all with a fork.
3. Pinch off some mixture, roll into 1 inch balls.
4. Place on a tray. Freeze 20 minutes. Serve.

Nutrition Values:

- Calories: 110.0
- Fat: 10.5g
- Carbs: 1.5g
- Protein: 2.3g
- Fiber: 0.2g
- Net Carbs: 1.3g

Sage and Cheddar Waffles

(Prep time: 10 minutes \ Cook time: 10 minutes\ 12 servings)

This delicious recipe is full of nutrition and you will like it.

Ingredients:

- ⅓ cup sifted coconut flour
- 3 tsp baking powder
- 1 tsp dried ground sage
- ½ tsp salt
- ¼ tsp garlic powder
- 2 eggs
- 2 cups canned coconut milk
- ¼ cup water
- 3 Tbsp melted coconut oil
- 1 cup shredded cheddar cheese

Preparation:

Preheat waffle iron.
1. In a bowl, combine the coconut flour, baking powder, sage, salt, garlic powder, and shredded cheese. Whisk together.
2. In a separate bowl, whisk the eggs. Add the coconut milk, water, melted coconut oil. Whisk briskly to combine. Add the dry ingredients to the wet. Stir until a batter forms.
3. Pour ⅓ scoop of batter onto waffle iron.
4. Close the iron. Cook until steam rises, 5-6 minutes.
5. Serve.

Nutrition Values:

- Calories: 213.97
- Fat: 17.21g
- Carbs: 9.2g
- Protein: 6.52g
- Fiber: 5.4g
- Net Carbs: 3.81g

Blueberry Mug Muffin
(Prep time: 1 minute\ Cook time: 1 minute\ 1 serving)

A sweet treat for one!

Ingredients:

- 1 Tbsp cream cheese
- 1 large egg
- 2 Tbsp vanilla whey protein
- ¼ tsp baking powder
- ⅛ tsp nutmeg
- ¼ cup fresh blueberries

Preparation:

1. Add the cream cheese to a large mug.
2. Heat in microwave 10 seconds. Stir until smooth.
3. Add the egg. Whisk with a fork to combine.
4. Add the whey powder, nutmeg, and baking powder to the mug. Mix well.
5. Add the blueberries. Stir.
6. Microwave 20 seconds. Cook at 15 second intervals if needed to cook longer.
7. Fork or spoon, can be used to enjoy this sweet treat.

Nutrition Values

- Calories: 242
- Fat: 15.1g
- Carbs: 6.3g
- Protein: 19.2g
- Dietary Fiber: 0.9g

Apple Tart

(Prep time: 30 minutes\ Cook time: 45 minutes\ 8 servings)

Apple tart is close to the heart. A classic for any diet routine.

Ingredients:

- 5 medium red apples
- ¼ cup sucralose based sweetener
- ¾ tsp cinnamon
- ⅛ tsp nutmeg
- 1 Tbsp unsalted butter
- 1 Cinnamon pie crust or pre-made pie shell

Preparation:

1. Cinnamon pie crust recipe is included in Breakfast section. Use that recipe or a pre-made pie shell.
2. Preheat oven to 350F.
3. Dice the apples into bite-size slices.
4. In a large bowl, combine the apple slices, sweetener, cinnamon, and nutmeg. Stir to coat the apple slices.
5. Spoon mixture into pie shell. Cut up the tablespoon of butter into small pieces. Place them on top of the apples.
6. Cover pie with top of pie crust.
7. Pierce top of pie in a few places to allow steam to escape.
8. Place on baking sheet. Bake 30 minutes.
9. Cover with aluminum foil and bake another 20 minutes, until apples are tender.
10. Cool the pie 30 minutes before slicing.

Nutrition Values

- Calories: 238
- Fat: 14.3g
- Carbs: 18.1g
- Protein: 8.2g
- Dietary Fiber: 3.1g

<u>**Berries With Chocolate Ganache**</u>
(Prep time: 10 minutes\ Cook time: 5 minutes\ 6 servings)

Waiting for a chocolate recipe? This recipe will fulfill all of your chocolaty dreams.

Ingredients:

- 1 cup strawberries
- 2 cups raspberries
- 2 cups blueberries
- ½ cup sugar-free chocolate chips
- ⅓ cup heavy cream
- ½ tsp pure vanilla extract

Preparation:

1. In a large bowl, combine the fruit. Stir.
2. Divide the fruit between 6 dessert bowls.
3. Boil a pot of water on medium heat. Place a glass bowl over the pot. Pour in the chocolate chips. Allow to melt. Stir in the cream. Remove from heat. Stir in the vanilla. Allow to cool slightly.
4. Pour over the fruit. Serve.

Nutrition Values

- Calories: 260
- Fat: 17.8g
- Carbs: 11.7g
- Protein: 2.3g
- Dietary Fiber: 7.4g

Caramelized Pear Custard

(Prep time: 10 minutes\ Cook time: 20 minutes\ 8 servings)

Caramelizing pears. Can you say drool?

Ingredients:

- 2 Tbsp butter
- 2 Tbsp Xylitol
- ¼ tsp ground cardamom
- 2 medium pears
- 3 eggs
- 2 egg yolks
- 2 cups heavy cream
- 1/8 cup sugar-free low calorie maple syrup
- ½ tsp rum
- 1 tsp pure vanilla extract

Preparation:

Preheating oven to 375F
1. Peel the pears. Slice them in half.
2. In a sauce pan, over medium heat, melt the butter. Add the rum, xylitol and cardamom. Stir well.
3. Add the pears to sauce pan. Cover with sauce. Cook 4 minutes per side.
4. Transfer the pears and sauce to a deep glass dish.
5. In a small bowl, whisk the eggs, egg yolks, maple syrup, heavy cream, and vanilla until fully combined and smooth. Pour mixture over pears.
6. Bake 20 minutes, until golden brown and the custard has set.
7. Remove from oven. Cool slightly before serving.
8. Using a pastry brush, lightly brush the pears with maple syrup. Serve.

Nutrition Values

- Calories: 310
- Fat: 27g
- Carbs: 7.6g
- Protein: 4.4g
- Dietary Fiber: 1.3g

Chocolate Brownie Drops

(Prep time: 15 mins\ Cook time: 15 mins\ 12 servings)

These brownie drops are both healthy and sweet.

Ingredients:

- ⅛ cup stone ground whole wheat pastry flour
- 2 Tbsp whole grain soy flour
- ¼ tsp baking powder
- ¼ cup unsweetened chocolate baking squares
- 6 Tbsp heavy cream
- 2 Tbsp unsalted butter
- 2 large eggs
- ¾ cup sucralose based sweetener

Preparation:

Preheat oven to 375F
1. Microwave the chocolate squares until almost melted. Add the butter. Stir until shinny. Set aside to cool.
2. Line a baking sheet with parchment paper.
3. In a large bowl, using an electric mixer, blend the butter until smooth. Add the sugar substitute. Blend again until smooth. Add the eggs, one at a time. Continue beating until smooth. Add the cooled chocolate to bowl. Continue beating.
4. In a separate bowl, whisk the flour, baking powder, and soy flour.
5. Pour in the flour mixture slowly. Beat until just combined.
6. Using a rounded spoon, spoon drops of batter onto the baking sheet.
7. Bake 5-6 minutes. Transfer to wire rack to cool. Serve.

Nutrition Values

- Calories: 104
- Fat: 9.4g
- Carbs: 3.9g
- Protein: 2.5g
- Dietary Fiber: 3.9g

Baked Pear Fans

(Prep time: 10 minutes\ Cook time: 40 minutes\ 4 servings)

While the recipe might seem bizarre, you will come to love the combination of these unique flavors.

Ingredients:

- 2 medium pears
- 1 Tbsp unsalted butter
- ¼ tsp black pepper
- ¼ tsp ginger
- ¼ tsp cinnamon
- 1 tsp tap water
- ¼ tsp pure vanilla extract

Preparation:

Preheat oven to 375F

1. You are going to make fans out of your pears. Make ¼ inch slices along the length of your half pear, starting ⅓ of an inch from the stem while cutting them all the way down to the bottom.
2. In a skillet, melt the butter. Add the lemon juice and water. Stir in the ginger, pepper, and cinnamon.
3. Place the pears in the skillet.
4. Cover with aluminum foil. Transfer skillet to oven. Bake 40 minutes. Turn the pears halfway through cooking.
5. Using a slotted spoon, transfer pears to serving plates.
6. Place skillet on stove. Stir in the vanilla. Simmer 1 minute.
7. Scoop the sauce over the pears. Serve.

Nutrition Values

- Calories: 80
- Fat: 3g
- Carbs: 11.5g
- Protein: 0.4g
- Dietary Fiber: 2.9g

Chocolate Frosty

(Prep time: 3 minutes\ Cook time: 0 minutes\ 1 serving)

A frosty! A chocolate one at that. Bring it on!

Ingredients:

- 2 Tbsp chocolate milk
- 2 Tbsp heavy cream
- 2 Tbsp sugar-free chocolate syrup
- ½ cup ice cubes

Preparation:

1. In a blender, combine the heavy cream, chocolate syrup, ice cubes. Blend until thick and smooth. Add a bit of chocolate milk for less thick consistency. Add more ice for a thicker consistency.
2. You could chill it for 20 minutes.

Nutrition Values

- Calories: 119
- Fat: 11.1g
- Carbs: 0.8g
- Protein: 1.6g
- Dietary Fiber: 1g

Ginger Flan

(Prep time: 180 minutes\ Cook time: 25 minutes\ 6 servings)

Unlike traditional pudding, this will give you a sweet taste and sensation of spice.

Ingredients:

- 3 egg yolks
- 2 egg
- 1½ cups heavy cream
- 1 cup tap water
- 8 packets sucralose based sweetener
- 1 tsp pure vanilla extract
- 3 tsp ground ginger

Preparation:

Preheat oven to 350F
1. Place a roasting pan on center shelf of oven. Fill to half with boiling water.
2. In a blender, combine the eggs, egg yolks, water, cream, sugar substitute, ginger, and vanilla. Blend until smooth.
3. Pass the sauce through a sieve. Pour into a 1-quart shallow baking dish.
4. Place the dish in the water bath in the oven. Bake 30-35 minutes.
5. Transfer to a cooling rack.
6. Once cooled, spray plastic wrap with non-stick cooking spray. Place it gently against the flan. Chill in the fridge 3 hours.
7. Once chilled, invert the baking dish and tap the flan onto a serving platter.

Nutrition Values

- Calories: 265
- Fat: 26g
- Carbs: 3.9g
- Protein: 4.6g
- Dietary Fiber: 0g

Coconut Cashew Bars

(Prep time: 10-15 minutes\ Cook time: 2 hours\ 8 servings)

A healthy nut bar you can make yourself. Satisfy a sweet tooth and healthy regime.

Ingredients:

- 1 cup almond flour
- 1 tsp cinnamon
- Pinch of salt
- ½ cup cashew nuts
- ¼ cup shredded coconut
- ¼ cup melted butter
- ¼ cup sugar-free maple syrup

Preparation:

1. In a large bowl, combine the flour, cinnamon, salt. Whisk briefly.
2. Smash the cashews. Add them with the coconut to the bowl.
3. Stir in the butter and maple syrup.
4. Line an 8x8 baking dish with parchment paper. Pour in the batter. Spread into an even layer.
5. Place in refrigerator. Chill 2 hours. Slice into bars.

Nutrition Values:

- Calories: 189.3
- Fat: 17.6g
- Carbs: 6.1g
- Protein: 4.4g
- Fiber: 2.1g
- Net Carbs: 4.0g

Choco Peanut Tart

(Prep time: 10-15 minutes\ Cook time: 30 minutes\ 4 servings)

Before the day ends, treat yourself with a tart.

Ingredients:

Crust

- ¼ cup flaxseed
- 2 Tbsp almond flour
- 1 Tbsp Erythritol
- 1 large egg (just need the egg white)

Middle Layer

- 4 Tbsp smooth peanut butter
- 2 Tbsp unsalted butter

Top Layer

- 1 medium avocado
- 4 Tbsp cocoa powder
- ¼ cup Erythritol
- ½ tsp pure vanilla extract
- ½ tsp cinnamon
- 2 Tbsp heavy cream

Preparation:

Preheat oven to 350F
1. Whisk the egg white.
2. In a large bowl, grind the flaxseed to a powdery consistency.
3. Add the almond flour, Erythritol. Stir in the egg white until crumbly.
4. Pour the mixture into a pie dish. Press in an even layer along bottom of pie dish. Bake for 8 minutes. Cool the crust completely before filling.
5. In a separate bowl, mash the avocado until smooth. Add the cocoa powder, Erythritol, cinnamon, vanilla extract, cream. Whisk until smooth.
6. In a separate bowl, melt the butter. Add peanut butter. Stir until smooth.
7. Pour the peanut butter batter in the pie dish. Spread in an even layer.
8. Pour the chocolate layer over the peanut butter layer. Smooth it out.
9. Refrigerator 1 hour.

Nutrition Values:

Calories: 304.8 Fat: 26.8g Carbs: 10.5g   Protein: 9.8g   Fiber: 6.6g

Brownies

(Prep time: 10 minutes\ Cook time: 20 minutes\ 8 large brownies)

Out of the hundreds of brownie recipes out there, this one is near perfect and delicious.

Ingredients:

- 1 Tbsp psyllium husk powder
- 2 cups almond flour
- 1 tsp baking powder
- ½ tsp salt
- ½ cup cocoa powder
- ⅓ cup Erythritol
- ¼ cup shredded coconut
- 2 large eggs
- ¼ cup maple syrup
- 2 Tbsp torani salted caramel

Preparation:

Preheat oven to 350F
1. Line an 8x8 baking pan with parchment paper. Grease with butter. Dust with cocoa powder.
2. In a large bowl, combine the husk powder, almond flour, baking powder, salt, cocoa powder, Erythritol, and shredded coconut. Whisk to combine.
3. In a separate bowl, whisk the eggs. Add the maple syrup, and salted caramel. Stir.
4. Fold the dry ingredients into the wet ingredients. Stir until just combined.
5. Bake 20 minutes.
6. Cool 30 minutes before slicing.

Nutrition:

- Calories: 258.1
- Fat: 23.7g
- Carbs: 10.4g
- Protein: 8.0g
- Fiber: 5.9g
- Net Carbs: 4.5g

Mini Vanilla Cloud Cupcakes

(Prep time: 10 minutes\ Cook time: 30-35 minutes\ 8 servings)

Ingredients:

Cupcakes

- 6 large eggs, room temperature
- 6 Tbsp cream cheese, room temperature
- ½ tsp cream of tartar
- 2 tsp pure vanilla extract
- ¼ cup granulated stevia/Erythritol mixture

Frosting

- ½ cup cream cheese, room temperature
- 2 Tbsp butter, room temperature
- ⅓ cup granulated stevia/Erythritol mix
- 1 Tbsp pure vanilla extract

Preparation:

Preheat oven to 300F
1. Separate the eggs yolks and egg whites.
2. Spray 2 muffin tins with non-stick cooking spray.
3. In a bowl, using an electric mixer, beat the cream cheese until smooth. Add the egg yolks one at a time. Stir in sweetener and vanilla extract until smooth batter.
4. In a separate bowl, whip egg whites until fluffy. Stir in cream of tartar.
5. Combine the egg whites with the egg yolk batter. Fold in gently until combined.
6. Using an ice cream scoop, fill the muffin tin cups ¾ full.
7. Place tin in oven. Bake 30-35 minutes, until toothpick comes out dry.
8. Place on cooling rack. Cool completely before icing.
9. In a bowl, combine the cream cheese and butter. Whip with electric mixer until smooth. Add the sweetener and vanilla. Whip until smooth.
10. Ice the cupcakes. Serve.

Nutrition Values:

- Calories: 347.9
- Fat: 30.8g
- Carbs: 6.9g
- Protein: 9.25g
- Fiber: 3.5g
- Net Carbs: 3.38g

Pumpkin Pecan Pie Ice Cream

(Prep time: 10 minutes\ Cook time: 10-15 minutes\ 4 servings)

We all scream for ice cream.

Ingredients:

- ½ cup cottage cheese
- ½ cup pumpkin puree
- 2 cups coconut milk
- 3 large egg yolks
- ⅓ cup Erythritol
- ½ tsp Xanthan gum
- 20 drops liquid Stevia
- 1 tsp pure maple extract
- 1 tsp pumpkin spice
- ½ cup toasted pecans, chopped
- 2 Tbsp salted butter

Preparation:

1. In a skillet, melt some butter. Toast the pecans. Set aside to cool.
2. In a separate bowl, combine the cottage cheese, pumpkin puree, coconut milk, egg yolks. Blend with electric mixer.
3. Stir in toasted pecans, xanthan gum, pumpkin spice, liquid stevia, maple extract.
4. Pour the mixture into an ice cream machine.
5. Churn according to instruction of ice cream machine. Serve.

Nutrition Values:

- Calories: 248.3
- Fat: 22.3g
- Carbs: 7.1g
- Protein: 6.5g
- Fiber: 2.9g
- Net Carbs: 4.3g

Amaretti Cookies

(Prep time: 10 minutes\ Cook time: 16 minutes\ 16 Cookies)

Fruit-filled cookies are downright addictive.

Ingredients:

- 1 cup almond flour
- 2 Tbsp coconut flour
- ½ tsp baking powder
- ¼ tsp cinnamon
- ½ tsp salt
- ½ cup Erythritol
- 1 Tbsp shredded coconut
- 4 Tbsp coconut oil
- 2 large eggs
- ½ tsp pure vanilla extract
- ½ tsp almond extract
- 2 Tbsp sugar-free jam

Preparation:

Preheat oven to 350F
1. Line a cookie sheet with parchment paper.
2. In a bowl, combine the almond flour, coconut flour, baking powder, cinnamon, salt, Erythritol. Whisk together.
3. In another bowl, add the coconut oil. Stir to soften it. Stir in one egg at a time. Add the vanilla. Stir until combined.
4. Add dry ingredients to wet ingredients. Stir until just combined.
5. Using a tablespoon, scoop cookie dough onto cookie sheet; 1 inch apart.
6. Dab your finger in water, and press an indent in the middle of the dough.
7. Bake 16 minutes.
8. Place on a cooling rack. Cool 30 minutes.
9. Add 1 teaspoon of jam to indent in cookie. Garnish with shredded coconut.

Nutrition Values:

- Calories: 85.7
- Fat: 7.9g
- Carbs: 2.5g
- Protein: 2.4g
- Fiber: 1.3g
- Net Carbs: 1.2g

Chocolate Dipped Macaroons

(Prep time: 10 minutes\ Cook time: 15 minutes\ 12 Macaroons)

Macaroons are really awesome for their gooey consistency and heart-melting flavor.

Ingredients:

- 1 cup shredded coconut
- 1 large egg white
- ¼ cup Erythritol
- ½ tsp almond extract
- Pinch of salt
- ½ cup sugar-free chocolate
- 2 Tbsp coconut oil

Preparation:

Preheat oven to 350F
1. Line a cookie sheet with parchment paper. Sprinkle the shredded coconut in a thin layer over the cookie sheet.
2. Bake 5 minutes. Watch the oven. Remove when golden brown.
3. Once the coconut is toasted, set aside. In a bowl, beat the eggs with an electric mixer until fluffy. Mix in the Erythritol and salt.
4. Add the cooled down toasted coconut to the batter. Stir well.
5. Drop 1 tablespoon of batter onto cookie sheet, 1 inch apart.
6. Bake 15 minutes, turn pan around. Bake another 15 minutes.
7. Remove from oven. Cool on pan 5 minutes, transfer to cooling rack to cool completely. Melt the chocolate.
8. Once cooled, dip macaroons in melted chocolate. Let them set 5 minutes.

Nutrition Values:

- Calories: 73.2
- Fat: 7.3g
- Carbs: 2.7g
- Protein: 1.0g
- Fiber: 1.7g
- Net Carbs: 1.0g

Baked Lemon Pork Chops
(Prep time: 15 minutes\ Cook time: 40 minutes\ 4 servings)

Make something which the whole family can enjoy.

Ingredients:

- 4 center cut pork chops, bone in
- 8 Tbsp tamari soy sauce
- 2 Tbsp Worcestershire sauce
- 2 garlic cloves, minced
- Juice from 1 lemon, Rind from half the lemon.
- 1 tsp canola oil
- ½ tsp fresh ground black pepper

Preparation:

1. In a small bowl, combine soy sauce, Worcestershire sauce, garlic, lemon juice, lemon rind, oil, and pepper. Whisk briskly to combine.
2. Pour mixture into a large Ziploc. Add pork chops. Massage marinade into chops. Chill 1-2 hours in the fridge.
3. Preheat oven to 375F.
4. Remove pork chops from baggie. Place in a deep baking dish.
5. Bake 15 minutes. Flip over. Bake another 20 minutes.
6. Let them rest 5 minutes before serving.

Nutrition Values

- Calories: 149
- Fat: 8
- Carbs: 4g
- Protein: 15.2g
- Dietary Fiber: 0.1g

Cali Mac & Cheese

(Prep time: 15 minutes\ Cook time: 20 minutes\ 6 servings)

This recipe is designed to save you from the horror of giving up mac and cheese.

Ingredients:

- 1 large cauliflower head
- 1 cup heavy cream
- 2 Tbsp cream cheese
- 1½ tsp yellow mustard
- 1½ cups shredded cheddar cheese + cheese for top
- 1 garlic clove, minced
- Pinch of salt and white pepper
- ¼ tsp original pepper sauce

Preparation:

Preheat oven to 375F
1. Break cauliflower into small pieces (medium shell pasta size). Cook until el dante.
2. Once cooked, drain water and pat the cauliflower dry.
3. In a medium sauce pan, heat the cream to a simmer.
4. Whisk in the cream cheese. Stir in mustard until combined.
5. Add shredded cheese, salt, white pepper, garlic. Stir until cheese melted.
6. Turn the heat off. Stir in the cauliflower pieces.
7. Pour mixture into deep baking dish. Top with grated cheese.
8. Bake 15 minutes, until cheese melted and golden brown.

Nutrition Values

- Calories: 320
- Fat: 27
- Carbs: 5.6g
- Protein: 11.4g
- Dietary Fiber: 3.6g

Avocado and Cheddar Omelet

(Prep time: 15 minutes\ Cook time: 20 minutes\ 6 servings)

Care to end your day the way you started it. Breakfast for dinner?

Ingredients:

- 1 tsp canola oil
- 4 large eggs
- ½ cup shredded cheddar cheese
- 1 avocado, sliced
- ½ cup salsa
- Pinch of salt and pepper

Preparation:

1. In a large bowl, add the eggs. Whisk them to combine. Stir in salt and pepper.
2. Heat oil in a large skillet.
3. Pour in egg mixture. Cook on one side. Flip to cook other side.
4. Spread cheese and avocado on one side. Flip in half.
5. Cook 1 minute to allow cheese to melt.
6. Top with salsa. Serve hot.

Nutrition Values

- Calories: 419
- Fat: 33.6g
- Carbs: 5.2g
- Protein: 20.8g
- Dietary Fiber: 5g

Yorkshire Pudding

(Prep time: 5 minutes\ Cook time: 35 minutes\ 8 servings)

Try this pudding straight out of Yorkshire.

Ingredients:

- 3 large eggs
- 1 cup whole milk
- ½ cup whole grain soy flour
- 1 Tbsp vital wheat gluten
- 1 tsp baking powder
- Pinch of salt
- ⅓ cup canola oil

Preparation:

Pre-heat oven to 450F
1. In a bowl, whisk the eggs and milk until combined.
2. In a separate bowl, combine the soy flour, wheat gluten, baking powder, and salt. Whisk.
3. Add dry ingredients to wet ingredients. Stir until smooth.
4. Grease an 8-inch square baking dish with oil.
5. Preheat baking dish 5 minutes in oven. Once oil is smoking, remove. Pour in batter. Bake 15 minutes.
6. Reduce temperature to 350F. Bake another 15 minutes, until golden brown.
7. Serve hot.

Nutrition Values

- Calories: 157
- Fat: 11.8g
- Carbs: 3.8g
- Protein: 9.2g
- Dietary Fiber: 0.5g

Stuffed Red Bell Peppers

(Prep time: 10 minutes\ Cook time: 45 minutes\ 4 servings)

Stuffed peppers are a meal all on their own.

Ingredients:

- 2 medium sweet red peppers
- ¼ cup feta cheese
- 8 cherry tomatoes
- ½ tsp ground thyme
- 2 Tbsp basil
- 2 Tbsp extra virgin olive oil

Preparation:

Preheat oven to 400F
1. Slice the tops off the peppers. Dice the good part. Remove seeds and ribs.
2. In a bowl, combine the tomatoes, feta cheese, thyme, basil, salt, and pepper. Drizzle in 1 tablespoon of the olive oil. Stir to coat ingredients.
3. Fill pepper shells with mixture.
4. Drizzle olive oil over deep glass baking dish.
5. Place peppers in, standing up. Cover with aluminum foil.
6. Bake 30 minutes. Remove foil. Bake another 15 minutes.

Nutrition Values

- Calories: 97
- Fat: 6.8g
- Carbs: 4.6g
- Protein: 3.2g
- Dietary Fiber: 1.9g

Braised Leeks and Fennel

(Prep time: 15 minutes\ Cook time: 45 minutes\ 8 servings)

Leeks and fennel on their own are fine. Braised with chicken broth and you have a meal!

Ingredients:

- 4 leeks, diced
- 1 fennel bulb, diced
- 1 cup chicken broth
- Pinch pepper
- 3 Tbsp unsalted butter
- 1 Tbsp fresh lemon juice
- ⅓ cup parsley, chopped

Preparation:

Preheat oven to 450F
1. In an 11 x 9 glass baking dish, add the leeks, fennel. Pour in the chicken broth. Season with pepper.
2. Cut up butter. Place over the ingredients. Cover baking dish with aluminum foil.
3. Bake 15 minutes. Remove from oven.
4. Stir in lemon juice. Garnish with parsley. Serve.

Nutrition Values

- Calories: 77
- Fat: 4.6g
- Carbs: 7.1g
- Protein: 1.3g
- Dietary Fiber: 1.8g

<u>**Maple and Sage Pumpkin**</u>
(Prep time: 10 minutes\ Cook time: 15 minutes\ 8 servings)

Pumpkins naturally taste pretty good, add some maple and sage and you have created an irresistible delight.

Ingredients:

- 1 pound of pumpkin
- ¼ cup shallots, chopped
- 1 Tbsp unsalted butter
- ¼ cup vegetable broth
- ½ cup sugar-free maple syrup
- ¼ tsp ground sage

Preparation:

1. Cube the pumpkin into ¾-inch pieces.
2. In a large skillet, melt the butter. Sauté shallots and pumpkin a few minutes.
3. Season with salt and pepper.
4. Sauté 8-10 minutes, until pumpkin is tender and slightly browned.
5. Pour in maple syrup. Add sage. Stir to coat pieces. Simmer 1 minute.
6. Serve hot.

Nutrition Values

- Calories: 26
- Fat: 1.2g
- Carbs: 3.5g
- Protein: 0.6g
- Dietary Fiber: 0.4g

Spicy Buffalo Cauliflower

(Prep time: 10 minutes\ Cook time: 45 minutes\ 4 servings)

A classic way eating your vegetables. Hide it with another flavor.

Ingredients:

- 1 large head of cauliflower
- 2 Tbsp light olive oil
- Pinch of salt and pepper
- 4 Tbsp buffalo wings sauce
- 3 tsp siracha sauce
- 2 Tbsp unsalted butter
- ½ cup crumbled blue cheese

Preparation:

Preheat oven to 375F
1. Line a baking sheet with parchment paper.
2. Cut the cauliflower into small florets.
3. Drizzle 1 tablespoon of the olive oil over the florets. Season with salt and pepper.
4. Spread the florets in a single layer on the baking sheet.
5. Bake 35-40 minutes.
6. As the cauliflower bakes, in a small saucepan combine the siracha and buffalo wings sauces together. Simmer 10 minutes.
7. Stir in the butter. Pull off the heat. Allow to cool to room temperature.
8. Once cauliflower cooked, toss them with the sauce. Pour onto serving platter. Garnish with crumbled blue cheese.

Nutrition Values

- Calories: 177
- Fat: 14.9g
- Carbs: 4.1g
- Protein: 5.3g
- Dietary Fiber: 4.2g

Asian Short Ribs

(Prep time: 45-60 minutes\ Cook time: 5-10 minutes\ 4 servings)

These might not be the BBQ ribs you are accustomed to, but give them a try and you won't
be disappointed.

Ingredients:

Ribs and Marinade

- 6 large short ribs
- ¼ cup soy sauce
- 2 Tbsp rice wine vinegar
- 2 Tbsp fish sauce

Spice Rub

- 1 tsp ground ginger
- ½ tsp onion powder
- ½ tsp minced garlic
- ½ tsp red pepper flakes
- ½ tsp sesame seeds
- ¼ tsp cardamom
- 1 Tbsp salt

Preparation:

1. In a small saucepan, combine rice wine vinegar, soy sauce, and fish sauce. Simmer 5
   minutes. Let it cool to room temperature.
2. Pour the marinade in a large Ziploc. Place ribs in the bag. Massage marinade into ribs.
   Let them rest for 60 minutes.
3. In a small bowl, combine ingredients of spice rub. Dump out marinade from the
   Ziploc. Place ribs in a large casserole dish. Coat ribs with spice rub.
4. Fire up your grill. Cook the ribs 3-5 minutes per side.
5. Serve hot.

Nutrition Values:

- Calories: 416.8
- Fat: 31.8g
- Carbs: 0.9g
- Protein: 29.5g
- Fiber: 0.0g
- Net Carbs: 0.9g

Italian Stuffed Meatballs

(Prep time: 10 minutes\ Cook time: 20 minutes\ 4 servings)

They might not look fancy but they taste divine.

Ingredients:

- 1½ pounds lean ground beef
- 1 tsp oregano
- ½ tsp Italian seasoning
- 2 garlic cloves, minced
- ½ tsp onion powder
- 3 Tbsp flaxseed meal
- Pinch of salt and pepper
- 3 Tbsp tomato paste
- 1 egg
- ½ cup green olives, sliced
- ½ cup mozzarella cheese, shredded
- 1 tsp Worcestershire sauce

Preparation:

Preheat oven to 400F
1. Line a baking sheet with aluminum foil.
2. In a large bowl, combine the ground beef, oregano, Italian seasoning, onion powder, salt, and pepper. Use your hands to blend the ingredients.
3. To that mixture, add tomato paste, egg, Worcestershire and flaxseed. Mix again.
4. Slice the green olives. Shred the cheese. Combine in a bowl together.
5. Take a pinch of ground beef mixture, flatten in your palm. Place a pinch of cheese and olives mixture in the middle. Wrap ground beef around it, form a ball. Makes approximately 20-30 meatballs, depending on size. If they are on the larger size, add a bit of cooking time.
6. Place meatballs on baking sheet, 1-inch apart. Bake 20 minutes.
7. Serve hot.

Nutrition Values:

- Calories: 593.5
- Fat: 44.8g
- Carbs: 6.0g
- Protein: 36.8g
- Fiber: 2.3g
- Net Carbs: 3.8g

<u>Nacho Chicken Casserole</u>

(Prep time: 10 minutes\ Cook time: 20 minutes\ 6 servings)

A unique South Western variation of Shepherd's Pie.

Ingredients:

- 2 Tbsp olive oil
- 2 pounds chicken thighs, boneless, skinless
- 1½ tsp chili seasoning
- ¼ cup cream cheese
- ¾ cup cheddar cheese x 2 (one for chicken mix, one for cauliflower mix)
- 1 cup green chilies and tomatoes
- ¼ cup sour cream
- 1 cup frozen cauliflower
- 1 jalapeno pepper, diced
- Pinch of salt and pepper

Preparation:

Preheat oven to 375F
1. Cut the chicken thighs in chunk-sized pieces.
2. In a skillet, heat the oil. Sauté the chicken until golden brown. Season with salt and pepper. Stir in the sour cream, cream cheese, cheddar cheese until melted. Add the green chilies and tomatoes, and jalapeno pepper. Stir well.
3. Cook the cauliflower. Using a blender, pulse the cauliflower until a mashed consistency. Add the shredded cheese. Stir well.
4. In a deep casserole dish, pour in a layer of the chicken mixture. Add the mashed cauliflower on top. Sprinkle with jalapeno peppers.
5. Bake 20 minutes. Remove from oven. Allow to set 5 minutes before slicing.
6. Garnish with fresh cilantro.

Nutrition Values:

- Calories: 426.0
- Fat: 32.2g
- Carbs: 5.9g
- Protein: 30.8gg
- Fiber: 1.7g
- Net Carbs: 4.3g

Oven Baked Turkey Leg

(Prep time: 10 minutes\ Cook time: 20 minutes\ 4 servings)

Just because it is not Thanksgiving does not mean you can't have turkey.

Ingredients:

- 2 medium turkey legs
- 2 Tbsp duck fat
- 2 tsp salt
- ½ tsp pepper
- ¼ tsp cayenne pepper
- ½ tsp onion powder
- ½ tsp dried thyme
- ½ tsp ancho chili powder
- 1 tsp liquid smoke
- 1 tsp Worcestershire sauce

Preparation:

Preheat the oven to 350F
1. Rinse the turkey legs with water, pat them dry.
2. In a small bowl, combine the liquid smoke, Worcestershire sauce. Stir.
3. In a separate bowl, combine the salt, pepper, cayenne pepper, onion powder, thyme, chili powder.
4. In a large skillet for the oven, melt the duck fat. Sear the turkey legs on all sides.
5. Place skillet in the oven. Bake 60-70 minutes. (Turkey leg internal temp: 180F)
6. Let turkey rest 5 minutes before serving.

Nutrition Values:

- Calories: 382
- Fat: 22.5g
- Carbs: 0.8g
- Protein: 44g
- Fiber: 0g
- Net Carbs: 0.8g

Slow Cooker Braised Oxtail

(Prep time: 15 minutes\ Cook time: 6-7 hours\ 3 servings)

Oxtails are extremely juice and tempting meals.

Ingredients:

- 1 Tbsp canola oil
- 2 pounds of Oxtail, bone in
- 2 cups beef broth
- ⅓ cup butter
- 2 Tbsp soy sauce
- 1 Tbsp fish sauce
- 3 Tbsp tomato paste
- 1 tsp onion powder
- 1 tsp minced garlic
- ½ tsp ground ginger
- 1 tsp dried thyme
- Pinch of salt and pepper
- ½ tsp guar gum

Preparation:

1. In a slow cooker, heat the beef broth, fish sauce, soy sauce, butter and tomato paste.
2. In a small bowl, combine the onion powder, ginger, thyme, salt, pepper. Coat the oxtail in seasoning.
3. In a skillet, on the stove, heat up the oil. Sear the oxtail on all sides. Transfer oxtail to slow cooker. Spoon the sauce over the oxtail. Cover.
4. Cook on low 6-7 hours. Check every hour to spoon the sauce over the oxtail.
5. Once cooked, remove the oxtail to rest. Turn up the heat on the slow cooker. Stir in guar gum to thicken the sauce.
6. Set the oxtail on a platter. Cover with the sauce. Serve.

Nutrition Values:

- Calories: 433.3
- Fat: 29.7g
- Carbs: 4.2g
- Protein: 28.3g
- Fiber: 1.0g
- Net Carbs: 3.2g

<u>Sushi</u>

(Prep time: 10 minutes\ Cook time: 10 minutes\ 3 servings)

A sushi carved out of cauliflower and cheese.

Ingredients:

- 1 cup cauliflower florets
- 1 package, 8 oz cream cheese, room temperature
- 1-2 Tbsp rice wine vinegar
- 1-2 Tbsp soy sauce
- 6 sheets of Nori
- 1 cucumber
- ½ an avocado
- 6 thin slices smoked salmon

Preparation:

1. Place the cauliflower in a blender. Pulse until rice-like consistency.
2. Slice the avocado thinly. Peel the cucumber. Cut in spears, removing middle. Place vegetables in fridge.
3. In a skillet, heat some oil. Sauté the cauliflower rice for 5 minutes. Stir in soy sauce. Set aside to cool down.
4. In a bowl, stir the cream cheese until smooth. Slowly stir in the rice wine vinegar until combined. Place in the fridge.
5. Cover a bamboo roller with saran wrap. Place a nori sheet on bamboo roller.
6. Spread cauliflower rice mixture over sheet. Add a piece of smoked salmon on top. Add a slice of avocado and a cucumber spear. Roll up the nori sheet. Continue making rolls until ingredients used.
7. Place in fridge until ready to eat.

Nutrition Values:

- Calories: 353.3
- Fat: 25.7g
- Carbs: 13.7g
- Protein: 18.3g
- Fiber: 8.0g
- Net Carbs: 5.7g

<u>Walnut Crusted Salmon</u>

(Prep time: 10 minutes\ Cook time: 15-20 minutes\ 2 servings)

A bite of this walnut-coated salmon is a bit of heaven.

Ingredients:

- ½ cup walnuts
- 2 Tbsp sugar-free maple syrup
- ½ Tbsp Dijon mustard
- ¼ cup fresh dill
- 2 x 3 oz salmon fillets
- 1 Tbsp olive oil
- Pinch of salt and pepper

Preparation:

Preheat oven to 350F
1. Place walnuts in blender. Pulse until crumbled.
2. Chop the dill. Transfer dill and walnuts to a bowl. Pour in the maple syrup. Stir in the Dijon mustard. Whisk the ingredients until combined.
3. Coat both sides of the salmon with the mixture.
4. In a large oven skillet, heat the olive oil. Sear salmon fillets per side for 3 minutes.
5. Transfer pan to oven. Bake 8-10 minutes. Serve hot.

Nutrition Values:

- Calories: 373
- Fat: 43g
- Carbs: 4g
- Protein: 20g
- Fiber: 1g
- Net Carbs: 3g

Blueberry Banana Smoothie
(Prep time: 10 \ Cook time: nil\ 1 serving)

For all the blueberry and banana lovers, this one is for you.

Ingredients:

- 3 Tbsp golden flaxseed meal
- 1 Tbsp chia seeds
- 2 cups vanilla coconut milk
- 10 drops liquid stevia
- ¼ cup blueberries
- 2 Tbsp MCT oil
- 1½ tsp banana extract
- ¼ tsp xanthan gum

Preparation:

1. Place all the ingredients in a blender.
2. Let it rest 5 minutes. Flaxseed will soak up some moisture.
3. Blend 1-2 minutes. Serve.

Nutrition Values:

- Calories: 264
- Fat: 25g
- Carbs: 10g
- Protein: 4g
- Fiber: 7g
- Net Carbs: 3g

Blackberry Chocolate Milkshake

(Prep time: 10 \ Cook time: nil\ 1 serving)

Craving dark chocolate? Whip up this milkshake.

Ingredients:

- 7 ice cubes
- 1 cup unsweetened coconut milk
- ¼ cup blackberries
- 2 Tbsp liquid stevia
- 12 drops xanthan gum
- 1-2 Tbsp MCT oil

Preparation:

1. In a blender, combine the ingredients.
2. Pulse until smooth. If too thick, add coconut milk.
3. Serve.

Nutrition Values:

- Calories: 338
- Fat : 34g
- Carbs: 11g
- Protein: 1g
- Fiber: 7g
- Net Carbs: 4g

Cucumber Spinach Smoothie

(Prep time: 10 \ Cook time: nil\ 1 serving)

Spinach and cucumber. A healthy snack.

Ingredients:

- 2 handfuls of baby spinach
- ½ cucumber, peeled, cubed
- 7 ice cubes
- 1 cup coconut milk
- 12 drops liquid stevia
- ¼ tsp xanthan gum
- 1-2 Tbsp MCT oil

Preparation:

1. In a blender, combine the ingredients.
2. Pulse until smooth. If too thick, add coconut milk.
3. Serve.

Nutrition Values:

- Calories: 335
- Fat: 33g
- Carbs: 7g
- Protein: 3g
- Fiber: 3g
- Net Carbs: 4g

Peanut Butter Caramel Milkshake

(Prep time: 10 \ Cook time: nil\ 1 serving)

A sweet treat to get you through the day, or night, or afternoon. Anytime is a good time for a milkshake.

Ingredients:

- 1 cup coconut milk
- 7 ice cubes
- 2 Tbsp smooth peanut butter
- 2 Tbsp SF torani salted caramel
- 1 Tbsp MCT oil
- ¼ tsp xanthan gum

Preparation:

1. Combine the ingredients in a blender.
2. Pulse until smooth. If too thick, add coconut milk.
3. Serve.

Nutrition Values:

- Calories: 366
- Fat: 35g
- Carbs: 9g
- Protein: 7g
- Fiber: 3g
- Net Carbs: 6g

Strawberry Milkshake

(Prep time: 10 \ Cook time: nil\ 1 serving)

A burst of strawberry in every sip.

Ingredients:

- ¾ cup coconut milk
- ¼ cup heavy cream
- 4 ice cubes
- ¼ cup frozen strawberries
- 1 Tbsp MCT oil
- ¼ tsp xanthan gum

Preparation:

1. Combine the ingredients in a blender.
2. Pulse until smooth. If too thick, add coconut milk.
3. Serve.

Nutrition Values:

- Calories: 367
- Fat: 43g
- Carbs: 3g
- Protein: 0g
- Fiber: 1g
- Net Carbs: 2g

Tropical Smoothie

(Prep time: 10 \ Cook time: nil\ 1 serving)

A refreshing burst in every sip.

Ingredients:

- ¾ cup unsweetened coconut milk
- 2 Tbsp golden flaxseed meal
- 1 Tbsp MCT oil
- 10 drops liquid stevia (optional)
- ¼ cup frozen mango
- ¼ cup frozen blueberries
- ¼ cup frozen banana

Preparation:

1. Combine the ingredients in a blender.
2. Pulse until smooth. If too thick, add more coconut milk.
3. Serve.

Nutrition Values:

- Calories: 352
- Fat: 31g
- Carbs: 8g
- Protein: 5g
- Fiber: 5g
- Net Carbs: 3g

In this chapter, I will be outlining a 3 weeks meal plan, which you could follow until you have reached a certain level of your goal. As for the part of meal plan, here is a quick overview as well- just for your convenience!

WHAT IS A MEAN PLAN?

You probably already know what a meal plan is but just to on the safe side; let's briefly discuss it. A meal plan is essentially a strategic blueprint of a diet plan that you are interested in following.

It contains everything from the nutrition values, products to purchase, what meal to eat, and when to eat, etc. Included here is a 4 week Keto Meal plan as a starting point of your keto diet journey.

SIX BENEFITS OF HAVING A MEAL PLAN

Having a total nutritional plan outlined has its benefits. Some of which are listed below

- It helps a lot in costs by allowing you to set up a rough estimate of your food budget earlier.
- It will enforce you to stick to the plan and eat as many healthy foods as possible
- Since you already know how much you are going to eat, you will not be wasting food either.
- You already know what you are going to cook ahead of time, so this will help you take a burden off your mind and mitigate your stress levels.
- Since you are aware of what you are going to do next, you won't be wasting time in choosing what to do. It will help to cook everything in time.
- It spices your life with different flavors as to avoid monotony in your meals.

These are just the tip of the iceberg. With a bit more research, you will be pleasantly surprised how much of a positive impact a meal plan can make in your daily life.

Week 1: Shopping List

- Salt
- Sucralose based Sweetener
- Cinnamon

- Unsalted butter
- Low carb baking mix
- Tap water
- Almond meal flour

- High fiber coconut flour (Organic)
- Cinnamon
- Baking powder

- Eggs
- Extra virgin olive oil
- Boneless pork loin
- Bone in pork loin chops
- Blue cheese
- Bacon
- Garlic
- Black ground pepper
- Fresh parsley
- Parmesan cheese
- Tomatoes
- Cilantro
- Red onion
- Jalapeno peppers
- Avocadoes
- Mayonnaise
- Lemon juice
- Basil
- Onion powder
- Celery salt
- Tilapia fillets
- Tamari soybean sauce
- Worcestershire sauce
- Canola oil
- Cayenne powder
- Yellow mustard seed
- Chicken wings (bone in)

Week 1: Meal Plan

Day One

(Totals: Calories: 625; Fat: 52.3g; Net Carbs: 15.5g; Protein: 53.9)

Breakfast:

Almond and Coconut Mug Muffin

(Calories: 207; Fat: 16.8; Carbs: 3.5g; Dietary Fiber: 3g; Protein: 9.7g)

Snack

Avocado Salsa(Calories: 71; Fat: 5.3g: Carbs: 3.3g; Protein: 1.1g)

Lunch

Broiled Parmesan Tilapia (Calories: 224; Fat: 12.8g: Carbs: 0.8g; Protein: 25.4g)

Dinner

Baked Lemon Pork Chops (Calories: 149; Fat: 8g: Carbs: 4g; Protein: 15.2g)

Dessert

Chocolate Brownie Drops (Calories: 104; Fat: 9.4g: Carbs: 3.9g; Protein: 2.5g)

Day Two

(Total: Calories: 1302; Fat: 75.5g; Net Carbs: 14.3g; protein: 50.1)

Breakfast:

Cinnamon Pie Crust With Fruit Filling(Calories: 193; Fat: 13.6g: Carbs: 2.5g; Protein: 14.8g)

Snack

Chicken Wings (Calories: 276; Fat: 18.5g: Carbs: 3.4g; Protein: 22g)

Lunch

Asian Beef Salad (Calories: 295; Fat: 13.3g: Carbs: 10.4g; Protein: 29.5gg)

Dinner

Cali Mac & Cheese (Calories: 320; Fat: 27g: Carbs: 5.6g; Protein: 11.4g)

Dessert

Baked Pear Flan (Calories: 80; Fat: 3g: Carbs: 11.5g; Protein: 0.4g)

Day Three

(Totals: Calories: 911; Fat: 70.8g; Net Carbs: 17g; Protein: 58.7g)

Breakfast:

Waffles (Calories: 193; Fat: 9; Carbs: 5.9; Dietary Fiber: 1.9g; Protein: 9.7g)

Snack

Artichoke with Three Cheeses (Calories: 57; Fat: 14g: Carbs: 3g; Protein: 4g)

Lunch

Crustless Quiche Loraine (Calories: 224; Fat: 12.8g: Carbs: 0.8g; Protein: 25.4g)

Dinner

Baked Lemon Pork Chops (Calories: 149; Fat: 8g: Carbs: 4g; Protein: 15.2g)

Dessert

Caramelized Pear Custard (Calories: 310; Fat: 27g: Carbs: 4.2g; Protein: 4.4g)

Day Four

(Total: Calories: 1033; Fat: 82.9g; Net Carbs: 19.6g; Protein: 48.3g)

Breakfast:

Almond and Coconut Mug Muffin (Calories: 207; Fat: 16.8g; Carbs: 3.5g; Protein: 9.7g)

Snack

Blackberry Peach Compote (Calories: 35; Fat: 0.2g: Carbs: 4.2g; Protein: 0.5g)

Lunch

Pan-Fried Tuna Patty (Calories: 367; Fat: 29.3g: Carbs: 2.4g; Protein: 24.2g)

Dinner

Cali Mac & Cheese (Calories: 320; Fat: 27g: Carbs: 5.6g; Protein: 11.4g)

Dessert

Chocolate Brownie Drops (Calories: 104; Fat: 9.4g: Carbs: 3.9g; Protein: 2.5g)

Day Five

(Totals: Calories: 1275; Fat: 88.7g; Net Carbs: 18.9g; Protein: 84.4g)

Breakfast:

Baked Egg & Asparagus (Calories: 471; Fat: 40g; Carbs: 5.6gg; Dietary Fiber: 4g; Protein: 20.8g)

Snack

Cinnamon Pie Crust With Fruit Filling(Calories: 193; Fat: 13.6g: Carbs: 2.5g; Protein: 14.8g)

Lunch

Broiled Parmesan Tilapia (Calories: 224; Fat: 12.8g: Carbs: 0.8g; Protein: 25.4g)

Dinner

Baked Lemon Pork Chops (Calories: 149; Fat: 8g: Carbs: 4g; Protein: 15.2g)

Dessert

Apple Tart (Calories: 238; Fat: 14.3g: Carbs: 6g; Protein: 8.2g)

Day Six

(Total: Calories: 1439g; Fat: 100.5g; Net Carbs: 11.9g; protein: 77.2g)

Breakfast:

Cinnamon Pie Crust With Fruit Filling

(Calories: 193; Fat: 13.6g: Carbs: 2.5g; Protein: 14.8g)

Snack

Indian Curry Chicken(Calories: 413; Fat: 22.1g: Carbs: 1g; Protein: 49.1g)

Lunch

Blue Cheese, Bacon, Chive Stuffed Pork Chops (Calories: 394; Fat: 26.3g: Carbs: 2g; Protein: 0.3g)

Dinner

Cali Mac & Cheese (Calories: 320; Fat: 27g: Carbs: 5.6g; Protein: 11.4g)

Dessert

Chocolate Frosty (Calories: 119; Fat: 11.5g: Carbs: 0.8g; Protein: 1.6g)

Day Seven

(Totals: Calories: 755; Fat: 52.3g; Net Carbs: 15.5g; Protein: 53.9)

Breakfast:

Almond and Coconut Mug Muffin

(Calories: 207; Fat: 16.8; Carbs: 3.5g; Dietary Fiber: 3g; Protein: 9.7g)

Snack

Avocado Salsa (Calories: 71; Fat: 5.3g: Carbs: 3.3g; Protein: 1.1g)

Lunch

Broiled Parmesan Tilapia(Calories: 224; Fat: 12.8g: Carbs: 0.8g; Protein: 25.4g)

Dinner

Baked Lemon Pork Chops (Calories: 149; Fat: 8g: Carbs: 4g; Protein: 15.2g)

Dessert

Chocolate Brownie Drops (Calories: 104; Fat: 9.4g: Carbs: 3.9g; Protein: 2.5g)

Week 2: Shopping List

- Salt

- Sucralose based Sweetener
- Cinnamon
- Unsalted butter
- Low carb baking mix
- Tap water
- Almond meal flour
- High fiber coconut flour (Organic)
- Cinnamon
- Baking powder
- Eggs
- Extra virgin olive oil
- Boneless pork loin chops
- Blue cheese
- Bacon
- Garlic
- Black ground pepper
- Fresh parsley
- Parmesan cheese
- Tomatoes
- Cilantro
- Red onion
- Jalapeno pepper
- Avocadoes
- Mayonnaise
- Lemon juice
- Basil
- Onion powder
- Celery salt
- Greek yogurt
- ketogenic peanut butter granola bar
- Strawberries
- Almonds
- Tilapia Fillets
- Tamari soybean sauce
- Worcestershire sauce
- Canola oil
- Center cut pork loin
- Cayenne powder
- Yellow mustard seed
- Bone-in chicken wings

Week 2: Meal Plan

Day One

(Total: Calories: 1252; Fat: 71g; Net Carbs: 18.9g; protein: 79.1g)

Breakfast:

Cinnamon Pie Crust With Fruit Filling(Calories: 193; Fat: 13.6g: Carbs: 2.5g; Protein: 14.8g)

Snack

Chicken Wings (Calories: 276; Fat: 18.5g: Carbs: 3.4g; Protein: 22g)

Lunch

Almond and Parmesan Crusted Tilapia (Calories: 344; Fat: 21.9g: Carbs: 6.6g; Protein: 29.3g)

Dinner

Cali Mac & Cheese (Calories: 320; Fat: 27g: Carbs: 5.6g; Protein: 11.4g)

Dessert

Chocolate Frosty (Calories: 119; Fat: 11.5g: Carbs: 0.8g; Protein: 1.6g)

Day Two

(Totals: Calories: 755; Fat: 52.3g; Net Carbs: 24.6g; Protein: 76.9g)

Breakfast:

Almond and Coconut Mug Muffin

(Calories: 405; Fat: 21; Carbs: 3.5g; Dietary Fiber: 3g; Protein: 9.7g)

Snack

ketogenic Peanut Butter Granola Bar with Yogurt and Strawberries Parfait

(Calories: 314; Fat: 9.5g: Carbs: 12.6g; Protein: 24.1g)

Lunch

Broiled Parmesan Tilapia (Calories: 224; Fat: 12.8g: Carbs: 0.8g; Protein: 25.4g)

Dinner

Baked Lemon Pork Chops (Calories: 149; Fat: 8g: Carbs: 4g; Protein: 15.2g)

Dessert

Chocolate Brownie Drops (Calories: 104; Fat: 9.4g: Carbs: 3.9g; Protein: 2.5g)

Day Three

(Total: Calories: 1252; Fat: 92.5g; Net Carbs: 18.9g; protein: 78.3g)

Breakfast:

Cinnamon Pie Crust With Fruit Filling(Calories: 193; Fat: 13.6g: Carbs: 2.5g; Protein: 14.8g)

Snack

Chicken Wings (Calories: 276; Fat: 18.5g: Carbs: 3.4g; Protein: 22g)

Lunch

Almond and Parmesan Crusted Tilapia (Calories: 344; Fat: 21.9g: Carbs: 6.6g; Protein: 29.3g)

Dinner

Cali Mac & Cheese (Calories: 320; Fat: 27g: Carbs: 5.6g; Protein: 11.4g)

Dessert

Chocolate Frosty (Calories: 119; Fat: 11.5g: Carbs: 0.8g; Protein: 1.6g)

Day Four

(Totals: Calories: 1196; Fat: 60.7g; Net Carbs: 24.8g; Protein: 77.1g)

Breakfast:

Almond and Coconut Mug Muffin

(Calories: 405; Fat: 21; Carbs: 3.5g; Dietary Fiber: 3g; Protein: 9.7g)

Snack

ketogenic Peanut Butter Granola Bar with Yogurt and Strawberries Parfait

(Calories: 314; Fat: 9.5g: Carbs: 12.6g; Protein: 24.1g)

Lunch

Broiled Parmesan Tilapia (Calories: 224; Fat: 12.8g: Carbs: 0.8g; Protein: 25.4g)

Dinner

Baked Lemon Pork Chops (Calories: 149; Fat: 8g: Carbs: 4g; Protein: 15.2g)

Dessert

Chocolate Brownie Drops (Calories: 104; Fat: 9.4g: Carbs: 3.9g; Protein: 2.5g)

Day Five

(Total: Calories: 1078; Fat: 91.6g; Net Carbs: 18.9g; protein: 79.1g)

Breakfast:

Cinnamon Pie Crust With Fruit Filling(Calories: 193; Fat: 13.6g: Carbs: 2.5g; Protein: 14.8g)

Snack

Chicken Wings (Calories: 276; Fat: 18.5g: Carbs: 3.4g; Protein: 22g)

Lunch

Parmesan Crusted Tilapia (Calories: 344; Fat: 21.9g: Carbs: 6.6g; Protein: 29.3g)

Dinner

Cali Mac & Cheese (Calories: 320; Fat: 27g: Carbs: 5.6g; Protein: 11.4g)

Dessert

Chocolate Frosty (Calories: 119; Fat: 11.5g: Carbs: 0.8g; Protein: 1.6g)

Day Six

(Totals: Calories: 1196; Fat: 60.7g; Net Carbs: 24.8g; Protein: 76.9g)

Breakfast:

Almond and Coconut Mug Muffin

(Calories: 405; Fat: 21; Carbs: 3.5g; Dietary Fiber: 3g; Protein: 76.9g)

Snack

ketogenic Peanut Butter Granola Bar with Yogurt and Strawberries Parfait

(Calories: 314; Fat: 9.5g: Carbs: 12.6g; Protein: 24.1g)

Lunch

Broiled Parmesan Tilapia(Calories: 224; Fat: 12.8g: Carbs: 0.8g; Protein: 25.4g)

Dinner

Baked Lemon Pork Chops (Calories: 149; Fat: 8g: Carbs: 4g; Protein: 15.2g)

Dessert

Chocolate Brownie Drops (Calories: 104; Fat: 9.4g: Carbs: 3.9g; Protein: 2.5g)

Day Seven

(Total: Calories: 1252; Fat: 92.5g; Net Carbs: 18.9g; protein: 108.4g)

Breakfast:

Cinnamon Pie Crust With Fruit Filling(Calories: 193; Fat: 13.6g: Carbs: 2.5g; Protein: 14.8g)

Snack

Chicken Wings (Calorie: 276; Fat: 18.5g: Carbs: 3.4g; Protein: 22g)

Lunch

Parmesan Crusted Tilapia (Calories: 344; Fat: 21.9g: Carbs: 6.6g; Protein: 29.3g)

Dinner

Cali Mac & Cheese (Calories: 320; Fat: 27g: Carbs: 5.6g; Protein: 11.4g)

Dessert

Chocolate Frosty (Calories: 119; Fat: 11.5g: Carbs: 0.8g; Protein: 1.6g)

Week 3: Shopping List

- Salt
- Sucralose based Sweetener
- Cinnamon
- Unsalted butter
- Low carb baking mix
- Tap water
- Almond meal flour
- High fiber coconut flour (Organic)
- Cinnamon
- Baking powder
- Eggs
- Extra virgin olive oil
- Boneless pork loin chops
- Blue cheese
- Bacon
- Garlic
- Black ground pepper
- Fresh parsley
- Parmesan cheese
- Tomatoes
- Cilantro
- Red onion
- Jalapeno pepper
- Avocadoes
- Mayonnaise
- Lemon juice
- Basil
- Onion powder
- Celery salt
- Greek yogurt
- ketogenic peanut butter granola bar
- Strawberries
- Almonds
- Tilapia fillets
- Tamari soybean sauce
- Worcestershire sauce
- Canola oil
- Cayenne powder
- Yellow mustard seed
- Chicken Wings

Week 3: Meal Plan

Day One

(Total: Calories: 1112; Fat: 296g; Net Carbs: 47.4g; protein: 75.6g)

Breakfast:

Cinnamon Pie Crust With Fruit Filling(Calories: 193; Fat: 13.6g: Carbs: 2.5g; Protein: 14.8g)

Snack

Apricot Apple Cloud (Calories: 9.9; Fat: 22.4g: Carbs: 25g; Protein: 1.5g)

Lunch

Simplified Barbeque Chicken (Calories: 330; Fat: 14g: Carbs: 2.6g; Protein: 45.6g)

Dinner

Cali Mac & Cheese (Calories: 320; Fat: 27g: Carbs: 5.6g; Protein: 11.4g)

Dessert

Berries with Chocolate Ganache (Calories: 260; Fat: 17.8g: Carbs: 11.7g; Protein: 2.3g)

Day Two

(Total: Calories: 1130; Fat: 80.1g; Net Carbs: 20.1; protein: 75.6g)

Breakfast:

Apple Muffin with Pecan Streusel (Calories: 242; Fat: 20.6g: Carbs: 5.3g; Protein: 7.5g)

Snack

Chicken Wings (Calories: 276; Fat: 18.5g: Carbs: 3.4g; Protein: 22g)

Lunch

Almond and Parmesan Crusted Tilapia (Calories: 344; Fat: 21.9g: Carbs: 6.6g; Protein: 29.3g)

Dinner

Baked Lemon Pork Chops (Calories: 149; Fat: 8g: Carbs: 4g; Protein: 15.2g)

Dessert

Chocolate Frosty (Calories: 119; Fat: 11.1g: Carbs: 0.8g; Protein: 1.6g)

Day Three

(Total: Calories: 1526; Fat: 87.8g; Net Carbs: 27.9; protein: 125.9g)

Breakfast:

Cinnamon Pie Crust With Fruit Filling(Calories: 193; Fat: 13.6g: Carbs: 2.5g; Protein: 14.8g)

Snack

ketogenic Peanut Butter Granola Bar with Yogurt and Strawberries Parfait

(Calories: 314; Fat: 9.5g: Carbs: 12.6g; Protein: 24.1g)

Lunch

Apricot Glazed Brisket (Calories: 358; Fat: 16g: Carbs: 1.3g; Protein: 47g)

Dinner

Avocado and Cheddar Omelet(Calories: 419; Fat: 33.6g: Carbs: 5.2g; Protein: 20.8g)

Dessert

Blueberry Cloud Muffin (Calories: 242; Fat: 15.1g: Carbs: 6.3g; Protein: 19.2g)

Day Four

(Total: Calories: 1088; Fat: 78.4g; Net Carbs: 21.2; protein: 72.7g)

Breakfast:

Almond and Coconut Mug Muffin (Calories: 207; Fat: 16.8g: Carbs: 3.5g; Protein: 9.7g)

Snack

Chicken Wings (Calories: 276; Fat: 18.5g: Carbs: 3.4g; Protein: 22g)

Lunch

Almond and Parmesan Crusted Tilapia (Calories: 344; Fat: 21.9g: Carbs: 6.6g; Protein: 29.3g)

Dinner

Yorkshire Pudding(Calories: 157; Fat: 11.8g: Carbs: 3.8g; Protein: 9.2g)

Dessert

Chocolate Brownie Drops(Calories: 104; Fat: 9.4g: Carbs: 3.9g; Protein: 2.5g)

Day Five

(Total: Calories: 689; Fat: 47.9g; Net Carbs: 25.1; protein: 44.8g)

Breakfast:

Cinnamon Pie Crust With Fruit Filling(Calories: 193; Fat: 13.6g: Carbs: 2.5g; Protein: 14.8g)

Snack

Avocado Salsa (Calories: 71; Fat: 5.3g: Carbs: 3.3g; Protein: 1.1g)

Lunch

Broiled Parmesan Tilapia(Calories: 224; Fat: 12.8g: Carbs: 0.8; Protein: 24.5g)

Dinner

Stuffed Red Bell Pepper

(Calories: 97; Fat: 6.8g: Carbs: 4.6g; Protein: 1.9g)

Dessert

Chocolate Brownie Drops (Calories: 104; Fat: 9.4g: Carbs: 13.9g; Protein: 2.5g)

Day Six

(Total: Calories: 1301; Fat: 94.2g; Net Carbs: 31.7; Protein: 85g)

Breakfast:

Protein Pancakes (Calories: 101; Fat: 9.9g: Carbs: 4.4g; Protein: 20g)

Snack

Chicken Wings (Calories: 276; Fat: 18.5g: Carbs: 3.4g; Protein: 22g)

Lunch

Almond and Parmesan Crusted Tilapia (Calories: 344; Fat: 21.9g: Carbs: 6.6g; Protein: 29.3g)

Dinner

Cali Mac & Cheese (Calories: 320; Fat: 27g: Carbs: 5.6g; Protein: 11.4g)

Dessert

Berries with Chocolate Ganache (Calories: 260; Fat: 17.8g: Carbs: 11.7g; Protein: 2.3g)

Day Seven

(Total: Calories: 1443; Fat: 108g; Net Carbs: 25.7g; Protein: 81.9gg)

Breakfast:

Cinnamon Pie Crust With Fruit Filling(Calories: 193; Fat: 13.6g: Carbs: 2.5g; Protein: 14.8g)

Snack

Chicken Wings (Calories: 276; Fat: 18.5g: Carbs: 3.4g; Protein: 22g)

Lunch

Almond and Parmesan Crusted Tilapia (Calories: 344; Fat: 21.9g: Carbs: 6.6g; Protein: 29.3g)

Dinner

Cali Mac & Cheese (Calories: 320; Fat: 27g: Carbs: 5.6g; Protein: 11.4g)

Dessert

Caramelized Custard (Calories: 310; Fat: 27g: Carbs: 7.6g; Protein: 4.4g)

Conclusion

Once again, I would like you to thank you for choosing this book and having the patience of reading it. I do hope you had as much fun reading and experimenting with the recipes as much I enjoyed preparing the book for you.

From now on, all you need to do is properly follow the rules of Ketogenic Diet and experiment with your very own meal plan!

Stay safe. Stay healthy. God Bless.